WHEN MUSCLE PAIN WON'T GO AWAY

The Relief Handbook for Fibromyalgia and Chronic Muscle Pain

GAYLE BACKSTROM
with
Bernard R. Rubin, D.O., F.A.C.P.
Professor of Medicine, Texas College of
Osteopathic Medicine

TAYLOR PUBLISHING COMPANY
DALLAS ■ TEXAS

PUBLISHED BY
Taylor Publishing Company
1550 West Mockingbird Lane
Dallas, Texas 75235

DESIGNED BY LURELLE CHEVERIE

Library of Congress Cataloging-in-Publication Data

Backstrom, Gayle.
When the muscle pain won't go away : the relief handbook for
Fibromyalgia and chronic muscle pain / Gayle Backstrom.
          p.   cm.
ISBN 0-87833-794-6 : $12.95
1. Fibrositis.   I. Title.
RC927.3.B33   1992
616.7'4—dc20   92-3289
                            CIP

Printed in the United States of America

10 9 8 7 6 5 4 3 2 1

■

WHEN MUSCLE PAIN WON'T GO AWAY

— ■ —

DEDICATED
TO MY GRANDMOTHER
DOVIE SMITH
AND
IN MEMORY OF
MY FRIEND
JEAN OLIVER

ACKNOWLEDGMENTS

I would like to thank each of the following individuals for their assistance on this book: Dr. David Teitelbaum and his office manager, Glenda Daniels, Fort Worth, Texas; Marty Cook, Executive Director, Arthritis Foundation, Northwest Texas Chapter, Fort Worth, Texas; Jacqueline King, Denton Regional Sports and Physical Therapy Center, Denton, Texas; Jean Judy, Assistant Professor, School of Occupational Therapy, Texas Women's University, Denton, Texas; Tom Hudgens, counselor, Texas Rehabilitation Commission, Denton, Texas; Dr. Robert Bennett, Oregon Health Sciences University, Portland, Oregon; Dr. P. Kahler Hench, Scripps Clinic & Research Foundation, La Jolla, California; Dr. Muhammad Yunus, University of Illinois College of Medicine, Peoria, Illinois; Dr. Frederick Wolfe and Mary Ann Cathey, Arthritis Center, Wichita, Kansas; Dr. Xavier J. Caro, University of California, Los Angeles; Dr. Don Goldenberg, Tufts University School of Medicine, Boston; Dr. Glen McCain, University of Western Ontario, London, Ontario; Dr. I. Jon Russell, University of Texas Health Sciences Center, San Antonio, Texas; Kristen Thorsen, *Fibromyalgia Network*, and Karen Samuelson, Fibromyalgia Association of Texas, Dallas. I also want to thank everyone who completed my fibromyalgia survey. Their responses helped me bring a personal element to this book.

I also want to thank those who kept me going during the work on the manuscript: Barbara Bartholomew, Linda Erickson, Joy Wright, Mary Vanecek, Bernice Latimer, Kathleen Moore, Dee Ann McFarlan, Billie Cantwell and, especially, Maurine Burnett.

Finally, a personal thanks to both of my editors at Taylor, Jim Donovan, who believed the time was right for this book, and Lorena Jones, who has been great to work with.

CONTENTS

WHAT YOU NEED TO KNOW   101

Over 30 of the most commonly asked
questions and their answers ■

A FINAL WORD   107

APPENDIX

Introduction

Over 20 years ago, at age 22, I was told that I had rheumatoid arthritis. As the years passed, that diagnosis was challenged as lab tests and X rays failed to confirm a rheumatoid arthritic condition. I was subsequently told that my pains were caused by systemic lupus erythematosis, bursitis, back strain, or more plainly, by symptoms that were all in my head. Finally, in the mid-1970s, I decided to get off the merry-go-round of doctors and tests. I planned to handle my pain by myself. I was fed up with the confusion and the response that I had to be psychologically creating my pain and stiffness because I looked too healthy and all the lab tests were negative.

I was able to stick to my decision with the help of aspirin and Tylenol until 1984, when a very mild horseback ride set off severe pain in my back and hips. It was then that I heard the word *fibrositis* for the first time. I was reassured that my pain would ease and that fibrositis was neither life threatening nor degenerative. I would just have to learn how to live with it.

While my life is not in danger, the other two statements have proven false. After being unable to work for several months, I took a job as a high school librarian and journalism teacher. The only way I was able to keep working was by spending every weekend and most of my evenings in bed. That lasted until 1986, when I developed severe chest pains. It took six months to determine that fibrositis was causing the pain, and by March, 1987, I had to quit my job.

Even teaching part-time as an adjunct for local colleges became too strenuous, yet the Social Security Administration decreed that as long as I made any effort to work, I was ineligible for disability payments. So the quality of my life has definitely been affected. I must use a wheelchair if I need to walk more than a few steps, and I cannot stand for any length of time beyond five minutes. I have recently obtained an electric scooter because I don't even have the energy to propel myself very far in the wheelchair. I can no longer work outside my home, where I must pace myself carefully to use the energy I do have to generate an income. Pain and fatigue limit my activities.

During a five-week hospital stay in early 1987, my doctor, Dr. Bernard Rubin, an associate professor at the Texas College of Osteopathic Medicine, talked with me about the lack of material on fibrositis that is available to the public. I began researching once I was out of the hospital and found that there were only a few articles even in rheumatology journals before 1982.

My search for a publisher to print a self-help book about *fibromyalgia* (the term that is now in use) proved fruitless, and I turned to writing romances. But I didn't give up on writing a book on fibromyalgia, and at intervals I sent out query letters to publishers and agents. In the spring of 1991, I made contact with Jim Donovan at Taylor Publishing in Dallas. Jim became as excited about the book as I was, and soon we were in business. Hence, the book you hold in your hand.

Although there are quite a number of terms in use, fibromyalgia (FM or FM syndrome) is now the generally accepted name. The syndrome has become well known. More and more doctors are recognizing FM, and more research is being conducted.

For myself, I was excited and relieved when a name was finally assigned to my pain and fatigue, allowing me to realize two things: I wouldn't die from some unknown and undiagnosed disease, and I wasn't crazy. It took a while longer before I learned the third thing: *I wasn't alone!*

Although the figures keep changing, about 5% of the American population suffers from FM. That's over 10 million Americans and doesn't include the millions of people with FM in other countries. One French researcher believed he had found a disease unique to his people. As we now know, that is not the case; FM appears worldwide and is one of the most common problems seen by rheumatologists.

I feel that I was extremely lucky to find Dr. Rubin. At our first meeting, he informed me that my chest pain was due to fibrositis. I desperately needed to get some relief from the unremitting pain, and I was very scared. At that office visit and in the years since, I have found him to be consistently knowledgeable about fibromyalgia and caring about me as a patient. Dr. Rubin has always been willing to talk with me about FM and its effects on me. He provided information about insurance companies, the Veterans' Administration, and Social Security benefits. He pointed me in the direction of the Texas Rehabilitation Commission, where I was able to get an adjustable chair that lets me sit at my computer longer and a laptop computer that I can use when I have to stay in bed.

I am glad Dr. Rubin agreed to work with me on this book, because, in this way, he can share some of his knowledge and caring with more people than he can ever see in his clinical practice. And I want to thank Dr. Rubin for his assistance. He was the first to urge me to write a book, when we began our patient-doctor relationship in December, 1986. In the years since then, he has given me encouragement and support in coming to terms with my fibromyalgia. He has worked with me within the limitations imposed by lack of health insurance and funds to progress as much as possible. I have a great deal of respect for him. Until I met him, the doctors I had seen did not know what I had, did not know what to do about it if they did have a name for it, or did not want to take the time with someone who has fibromyalgia. It is because of Dr. Rubin that I have been able to write *When Muscle Pain Won't Go Away*. He believes that the individual should take responsibility for his or her care and has shown me how to do that. I wish for you the same type of care from your doctor.

This book is not intended to take the place of a physician. If you have not been diagnosed with fibromyalgia, but think that you might have it, you should consult a physician.

Here you will find a brief history of FM, an explanation of the diagnostic criteria recently established by the American College of Rheumatology for the classification of fibromyalgia, information about associated conditions, and theories on possible causes. We will look at various modes of treatment and ways you can work, as an active partner with your doctor, to live with FM.

I try to avoid using the word patient throughout this book, relying on words such as individual or person instead. I do this because I believe we should focus on the positive rather than the negative. By referring to people as patients, the emphasis is focused on the illness, not the person. The word patient also implies vulnerability and loss of control. People with FM must focus on what they can do in spite of their FM. Each individual must take control of his or her life and live each day to the best extent possible. I urge you to learn the information in this book and to use it to overcome the limitations and troubles FM has brought to your life. Good luck and, remember, you can live with fibromyalgia and still have a rich and rewarding life.

What Is Fibromyalgia and Why Do I Hurt All the Time?

"I hurt all over, just like the flu but much worse."

"I can't do the things I used to do, like running or walking through an amusement park. My kids tell me I'm no fun to be around anymore."

For most people, coping with fibromyalgia syndrome has been a frustrating, painful experience. They have faced doctors who discounted any problems unconfirmed by laboratory tests or X rays. Some of them have doctors who are reluctant to admit that their problems are bewildering and whose solution is to refer them to a psychiatrist or psychologist.

Until recently, people with fibromyalgia had the best chance of getting a correct diagnosis if they saw a rheumatologist, but even many rheumatologists either were not well informed about FM or chose not to spend the time necessary to understand and work on the problem. Because there is no magical cure for FM, treatment must focus on the symptoms and must come from a partnership between doctor and individual.

Education is the first step toward achieving relief. Once you learn as much as you can about FM, you will have more control over your well-being and your treatment. In fact, learning the basic information about FM may prevent you from having to undergo unnecessary tests and treatments.

One 57-year-old woman went to 14 different doctors and 2 physical therapists and spent over $40,000 trying to find relief. She also had four unnecessary minor surgeries, one of which left her in more pain than she experienced before the surgery. Another woman, 48 years old, was told that she didn't know how to be happy because of her childhood and that unhappiness was the cause of her constant pain.

Just what is fibromyalgia and why do people with it have such a hard time obtaining a diagnosis? Why do they often go from doctor to doctor or face suggestions that it is all in their minds?

Fibromyalgia has been known by many names since it was first identified by the medical community. Depending on which authority you believe, that could reach back to the beginning of this century or even extend back to ancient times. FM is characterized by widespread *musculoskeletal* (muscles and bones of the body) pain, stiffness, and fatigue. It occurs more often in women than in men, and the average age of those who get FM is mid-to late 40s. Yet it can also affect children and older people. Some people can recall a specific incident or illness that marked the beginning of their problems. But for others, the pain and discomfort progressed so gradually that they can't pinpoint the condition's onset. For some people, FM presents only minor problems, while it has changed other people's entire lives. There are those who have adjusted to the changes brought on by FM, and then there are others who are angry, confused, and frustrated. They are frustrated not only by the symptoms but also by the responses and attitudes of members of the medical profession who do not recognize FM or who cannot or will not spend the time necessary to treat it.

The first step in treating any health problem is arriving at a correct diagnosis and progressing into a mode of treatment. Fibromyalgia is finally becoming known beyond the realm of rheumatology, so the odds that those with FM will secure a correct diagnosis are constantly improving. Various modes of treatment are available, but for everyone the first step is learning about the history of fibromyalgia, its symptoms, and the existing options for treatment.

Dr. Hugh Smythe, professor and head of the Rheumatic Diseases Unit at the Wellesley Hospital in Toronto, covered fibrositis in his chapter on nonarticular rheumatism in an arthritis textbook in the early 1960s. Smythe is generally regarded as the person who brought fibrositis into the spotlight, sparking research on the elusive syndrome in the late 1970s.

Dr. Smythe began to work with Dr. Harvey Moldofsky, the University of Toronto and also of the Wellesley Hospital, who was exploring the relationship between sleep patterns and the pain of fibrositis. Dr. Moldofsky's research showed the intrusion of alpha waves into stage-four, or non-rapid-eye-movement restorative, sleep of people with FM, which disrupted that essential stage of sleep. Except for two subjects who were considered aerobically fit, the symptoms of fibrositis developed in the healthy test subjects when their sleep was similarly disturbed; when they were allowed undisturbed sleep, their symptoms disappeared.

Of particular interest to other researchers was the presence of *tender points*. They are found in specific spots throughout the body; most people with fibromyalgia are not aware of their presence. Dr. Smythe was the first to designate the presence of tender points as a symptom of FM, but Dr. Moldofsky's experiments showed they could be reproduced when sleep was disrupted. Finally, a tie was identified between a sleep disorder and the uncontrollable pain of the tender points.

The terms fibromyalgia and fibrositis were used almost interchangeably until the late 1980s, when it was recommended that the term fibrositis be dropped. *Fibro* refers to the muscles, but *itis* refers to inflammation, and no one has been able to detect any inflammation in the muscles.

Other names include but are not limited to myofascial pain syndrome, muscular rheumatism, primary fibromyalgia, secondary or concomitant fibromyalgia, and tension *myalgia* (pain in the muscles). Some doctors still use some of these terms, which only adds to the confusion. Throughout the 1980s many doctors and researchers set their own criteria for diagnosing fibromyalgia. This created confusion and problems, including the needless replication of research studies. Different physicians required various numbers of tender points to be painful to confirm an FM diagnosis, as well as the presence or absence of other health problems.

Primary fibromyalgia was considered to be the problem when no other illness or rheumatic condition could be found. When a disease such as rheumatoid arthritis, osteoarthritis, or lupus was discovered, the diagnosis became *secondary fibromyalgia*. All of this led the American College of Rheumatology to create a criteria committee in 1989 to formally identify and declare the syndrome's characteristics. Researchers from 16 medical centers in the United States and Canada met to consider establishing definitive criteria for diagnosing fibromyalgia. "Widespread pain" had to be defined, and a host of miscellaneous symptoms and associated conditions also needed clarification. Representatives from the research centers evaluated all of the guidelines they had used at their centers and finally developed two criteria for diagnosing the syndrome. The American College of Rheumatology published the definitive criteria for the classification of fibromyalgia in 1990.

It was recognition of the tender points that helped eliminate fibromyalgia's image as a psychological catchall. The American College of Rheumatology determined that those suffering from FM have at least 11 out of 18 designated tender points, symmetrically located throughout the body, that elicit pain when pressed by the examiner, while control points located elsewhere on the body do not. Areas of tenderness in those with FM are not painful in control subjects. There are other symptoms and accompanying conditions that occur in fibromyalgia but are not always present in every person. The Criteria Committee decided that although these symptoms and conditions may be common, widespread pain and tender points were more common, showing up in almost

THE AMERICAN COLLEGE OF RHEUMATOLOGY'S CRITERIA FOR CLASSIFYING FIBROMYALGIA

1. History of widespread pain

   Pain is considered widespread when all of the following are present: pain in the left side of the body, pain in the right side of the body, pain above the waist, and pain below the waist. In addition, *axial skeletal* pain (pain in the *cervical* spine [neck], chest, *thoracic* spine [upper back], or lower back) must be present. In this definition, shoulder pain and buttock pain qualify as pain for each involved side. Lower back pain is considered lower segment pain (below the waist).

2. Pain in 11 of 18 tender point sites upon *digital palpation* (pressure applied with the fingers)

   In other words, pain, on digital palpation performed with an approximate force of 4 kg, must be present in at least 11 of the 18 designated tender point sites. For a tender point to be considered positive, the subject must feel pain, not tenderness, upon palpation.

   For classification purposes, fibromyalgia will be diagnosed if both criteria are satisfied. Widespread pain must have been present for at least three months. The presence of a second clinical disorder does not change the diagnosis of fibromyalgia.

Courtesy of Dr. Frederick Wolfe. Reprinted with permission from *Arthritis and Rheumatism*.

100% of those studied, and therefore must serve as the basis for a fibromyalgia diagnosis.

The committee also voted to drop the guidelines for determining the differentiation between primary and secondary fibromyalgia. Whether another rheumatic condition or illness was present was not important; they decided that fibromyalgia, on either level, should be recognized and treated.

In addition to the committee's criteria for diagnosis, Dr. Frederick Wolfe, a member of the committee from the University of Kansas School of Medicine, devised a four-part theory that organizes the symptoms and findings on FM. He considered the first two symptoms (widespread pain and tender points) to be the core features. But there were other aspects of the syndrome that Dr. Wolfe believed to be significant and worth recognition. Characteristic features occur in about 75% of those with FM. These include fatigue, nonrestorative sleep, and morning stiffness. Common features occur in about 25% of those with FM and include irritable bowel syndrome, Raynaud's phenomenon, (a condition in which the arteries of the fingers are unusually reactive and become spastic when the hands are cold) headaches, and other problems. Finally, there are coexisting rheumatic conditions such as rheumatoid arthritis, osteoarthritis, systemic lupus erythematosis, and others that are present in addition to fibromyalgia.

Modulating Factors

Just as many illnesses wax and wane, so does fibromyalgia. Some days are very bad, and others are fairly good. Sometimes the reason for this is difficult to find. At other times the factors that can make the symptoms worse are quite clear. Some of them commonly affect other rheumatic conditions such as rheumatoid arthritis and osteoarthritis. The weather is a primary factor. Cold, damp weather makes the aching worse and increases the amount of pain. Those with FM aren't too different from arthritis sufferers who have a bad knee that predicts the weather. Very hot weather can leave some feeling almost ill, although the reason is not certain. Sitting in the draft from an air conditioner can also increase the pain of FM, and many people find they cannot sleep with an air conditioner blowing directly into the bedroom. This sensitivity to both heat and cold has been noted in many studies.

Physical and mental fatigue can increase the pain level, as well. It is not unusual to experience a flare-up of pain after physical exertion. This can become a cycle that is hard to break. Increased activity causes increased pain, but if there is no way to take the necessary rest and you must continue to work, more pain follows. You might be able to get away with working six or seven hours at a time, but if you continue to push and work every day, your pain level may also continue to increase. You need to give yourself time enough to rest if at all possible. While excess physical activity aggravates the symptoms for some people with fibromyalgia, everyday activities require enough physical stress to create pain.

On the other side of the coin, physical inactivity can cause FM symptoms to worsen. So some physical exercise is necessary in moderation. The longer you go without some sort of exercise, the harder it becomes to exercise at all and the more deconditioned you become. The wise course is to achieve a careful balance between exercising enough to increase your aerobic fitness and produce more natural *endorphins* (the body's painkillers) and not exercising so much that your body becomes antagonized.

A poor night's sleep will also generate more pain and fatigue. This may sound strange when disturbed sleep has already been named as one of the problems of fibromyalgia. But even beyond that intrusion into the stage-four sleep, there are additional factors that can prevent you from getting enough rest. They can include everything from sleeping on a mattress that does not provide sufficient support to having the room temperature too cold.

One of the other factors that has a strong impact on FM and its symptoms is stress. This is not surprising when we know that stress affects everything from blood pressure to gastrointestinal problems. However, just as negative stress can have an impact, so can positive stress. Sometimes our bodies don't know the difference between positive and negative excitations, giving the same physical response for both. The recognition that stress can make FM symptoms worse does not mean that it is psychological. We are finding more and more evidence that the link between the mind and the body is a much stronger one than we thought. What affects the mind affects the body. Stressors can include anything from financial difficulties to an unhappy marriage, from a troublesome job to a high neighborhood crime rate.

MODULATING FACTORS FOR FIBROMYALGIA

Aggravating Factors	Relieving Factors
Cold or humid weather	Warm, dry weather
Nonrestorative sleep	Hot showers or baths
Physical/mental fatigue	Restful sleep
Excess physical activity	Moderate activity:
Physical inactivity	stretching exercises
Anxiety/stress	and massage

Courtesy of Dr. P. Kahler Hench. Reprinted with permission from *Rheumatic Disease Clinics of North America*.

In his book *Chronic Muscle Pain Syndrome*, Dr. Paul Davidson asserts that stress is the cause of "fibrositis" and if people with FM would only acknowledge this and work to better handle their stress, their fibrositis would go away. He describes a "fibrositic personality" and discusses how it prompts the body to react with fibrositis. Dr. Davidson's theory is not supported by documentation in medical journal articles. While it is generally accepted that stress can intensify the symptoms, the concept of a fibrositic personality has been disputed by a number of researchers. Dr. Davidson says, "Fibrositis symptoms can leave and never return if you are able to deal adequately with the causes. If you do not or cannot, however, the symptoms may return." While there are cases of remission among people with FM, lasting anywhere from two months to twenty years, most researchers have found that fibromyalgia symptoms generally remain, regardless of the method of treatment used.

If the above factors make the symptoms worse, is there anything that can make them better? Yes. Those with FM typically find that their symptoms are eased by warm, dry weather, hot showers or baths (or a session in a hot tub), restful sleep, and participation in moderate activity including stretching exercises and massages.

Coexisting Rheumatic Conditions

It is possible for a person to have fibromyalgia and another rheumatic condition at the same time. Before the American College of Rheumatology's Criteria Committee voted to eliminate the terms, fibromyalgia was classified as primary or secondary (concomitant). When no other rheumatic condition was found, the individual was diagnosed with primary fibromyalgia. Those who had another rheumatic condition were diagnosed with secondary, or concomitant, fibromyalgia. The most common rheumatoid conditions occurring with fibromyalgia were rheumatoid arthritis, osteoarthritis, tendonitis-peritendonitis, lupus, and lower back pain. Often when an individual had another condition, the fibromyalgia was almost disregarded. Fibromyalgia can often make another medical condition more severe, and treatment should be handled accordingly.

Functional Disability

There is a percentage of individuals who do develop a functional disability. At this time, there aren't any clear indications of how large that percentage is. Figures range from 5% to 22%. There are also a number of women with FM who do not work outside the home and as a result are not reported as disabled, but who have difficulty managing to maintain their households.

There are several key points worth noting. First, if at all possible, you should continue to work, if you are employed, for as long as you can. This is not only advisable because of the money you will earn—although that is important regardless of whether you are single or married—but also because insurance coverage, or the lack of it, can have a major impact on your condition. Money worries and the inability to pay for medical care can add a good deal of stress to an already overtaxed system.

However, we must deal with reality. Sometimes reality gives you no choice, and you find you must quit your job. If you are financially able to do so, even for a short period, this may give you time to break the pain cycle. Few families can manage when they lose one partner's income. But don't give up with the attitude that you'll never be able to work again.

One woman in her late 20s quit her job and took six weeks to rest and have physical therapy. Her symptoms eased, and she began writing a newsletter for people with fibromyalgia. Quite often a change in the type of job or the number of hours worked will help. If you need retraining, ask your doctor to refer you to the state vocational rehabilitation agency. The names may vary, but there should be an agency in every state.

If you are forced to quit work, make sure you take advantage of the new COBRA law. This is a federal law that requires your company and its insurance provider to allow you to pay for your insurance coverage for up to 18 months after you leave a job. The purpose is to provide a transition between insurance companies when you move to a new job. You must pay for the coverage, which cannot be any different than what you had as an employee. The cost includes a minor administrative fee—something in the neighborhood of 2%—but, other than that fee, the cost cannot be more or the benefits fewer.

Quite often, people with FM get caught up in the medicolegal system. Their symptoms may have begun with a traffic accident or a work-related injury. They generally end up on a merry-go-round that drags them from lawyer to workman's compensation doctor to their own doctor. Because tests and X rays often do not confirm an FM diagnosis, resulting in a lack of verifiable documentation, the chances of receiving some form of compensation may be slim. If you have been successful, great. If you are considering such action, make an informed decision about what to do based on your doctor's advice and your specific situation. Just be aware that as long as the process drags out, the stress will affect you adversely.

Do not assume that because you have been diagnosed with fibromyalgia that you will become totally disabled. Be aware that although this book covers all phases of FM, only you and your doctor know what phase you are at. And there is no guarantee that because you have severe symptoms in the beginning that they will stay that severe. Fibromyalgia presents a puzzle that is still so poorly understood that the only thing many people know for sure is that they can't know what to expect.

How Many People Have FM and How Many More May Get It?

Who develops fibromyalgia, and what can they expect in terms of the future? There are some answers to these questions, but you must understand that there is still a great deal about FM that even the experts don't know. Most of the studies that have been conducted over the last 12 to 15 years have been done primarily by rheumatologists. The very nature of their practice has defined some of the parameters.

People with FM who have spent months, if not years, searching for medical help are often those with severe symptoms. They have seen their family doctors, internists, and perhaps orthopedists or neurologists. They have continued to search because they have failed to find anyone who can give them an accurate diagnosis and a successful treatment. One woman says that she's had so many diagnoses that she's still afraid to trust the one for FM.

The main point is that those people who took part in many of the studies may have more severe problems than those in the general population. Up to this time, only one study has been conducted in the community at large, where it can be assumed that there are a number of people who have fibromyalgia but who have not sought medical help for it. Just how many people are there who have FM? We can only guess.

The estimates have been increasing over the last ten years. In the early journal articles, figures generally ran between three and six million. By the late 1980s the figure had increased to nearly 10 million Americans. Remember that everyone did not agree on the same criteria for diagnosis, and most figures did not include anyone who had another rheumatic condition such as rheumatoid arthritis, lupus, or even osteoarthritis, which almost everyone gets as they grow older.

Now that the American College of Rheumatology has established criteria for classifying FM and refuses to use the secondary or concomitant classification, we should be getting a clearer picture. In 1989 Dr. Robert Bennett, at the Oregon Health Sciences University in Portland, Oregon, and Dr. Don Goldenberg, at the Newton-Wellesley Hospital in Newton, Massachusetts, estimated that FM affects about 5% of the American population, or about 10 million people in the United States. They also estimated that 15% to 40% of the cases referred to American rheumatologists are FM or FM related. FM has become one of the three most common conditions seen by rheumatologists.

Who Gets Fibromyalgia?

Studies up to this point have focused more on the symptoms than on the demographics of those with FM. Even when researchers did gather personal information, it was often affected by the location of the clinic. Some had an older patient group or a more rural community to draw from. Most reports indicate that women are more likely to get fibromyalgia than men. On the average, fibromyalgia usually strikes individuals in their 40s to 50s, but the onset can occur anywhere from early adolescence to the 30s and 40s. Remember these are only averages; there will be some individuals who get FM in their 20s and others in their 60s or 70s. Mary Ann Cathey and Dr. Frederick Wolfe, who formed one of the few groups to study demographics, found the FM individuals they studied to have just a bit more education and to make just above the average income for a Kansas family.

No studies have been conducted regarding ethnic groups or occupations. But it must be remembered that research takes money, and many of the foundations or organizations that fund such research generally have more requests than they can meet. FM is the new kid on the block and is only now becoming recognized as a legitimate subject for study. Even when doctors get funding for research, the first objective is to find the cause or causes and develop a successful mode of treatment, rather than to look at who does or can develop FM.

How does it start? Some people can remember an accident or an emotional trauma that seemed to cause their muscular aches and pain, and some believe it began with a flu-like illness that never went away. For others though, the syndrome progressed so gradually that there is no date they could point to with certainty as the beginning. Some can remember having such aches or recurring "growing pains" even as children.

Myofascial pain syndrome has often been confused with fibromyalgia, because it has "trigger points" that cause pain. There is a significant difference between tender points and trigger points, although the terms were used almost interchangeably in early research. Unlike the tender points of FM, however, pressing trigger points causes pain to register in another spot, usually in deep muscle. Myofascial pain is a localized condition, occurring in one particular area, such as a shoulder or hip. During the 1980s, many people with FM were diagnosed with myofascial pain because they complained about one area—the area that seemed to hurt the most. However, if their doctors questioned them closely, other areas were also found to be painful. Some theories contend that fibromyalgia is myofascial pain gone too long untreated.

At this point no one knows exactly why someone develops FM or why it develops differently in different individuals. One theory suggests that some people are genetically disposed to the development of FM but cannot explain why certain events or stressors provoke it.

What Can I Expect?

Fibromyalgia is a chronic condition. There is no magic pill that will cure it. But it is important to remember that it is not deforming like rheumatoid arthritis, and it is not life threatening. It is a condition that fluctuates, with good days and bad days, although it remains remarkably stable over time. There is also the chance that it will go into remission, which is considered to be a period of at least two months without symptoms. Remission can last anywhere from two months to twenty years. The amount of relief from a particular mode of treatment will vary from patient to patient and even within each patient, due to the number of

DOCTOR'S QUESTIONNAIRE FOR DETERMINING THE SEVERITY OF YOUR FM AND CHARTING YOUR PROGRESS

Were you able to:	Always	Most times	Occasionally	Never
Do shopping	0	1	2	3
Do laundry with a washer and dryer	0	1	2	3
Prepare meals	0	1	2	3
Wash dishes/cooking utensils by hand	0	1	2	3
Vacuum a rug	0	1	2	3
Make beds	0	1	2	3
Walk several blocks	0	1	2	3
Visit friends/relatives	0	1	2	3
Do yard work	0	1	2	3
Drive a car	0	1	2	3

Courtesy of Dr. Robert M. Bennett, Carol S. Burckhardt, R.N., Ph.D., and Sharon R. Clark, R.N. Reprinted with permission from the *Journal of Rheumatology*.

variables, some of which are not clearly understood, that are involved in FM. Sometimes the relief will be only temporary and a new method of treatment must be sought.

At this time, there is no sure method of treatment that is guaranteed to bring about permanent remission. Although this is a reality that must be confronted, it does not mean that there is no hope for improvement. But first it is important that you accept that fibromyalgia has become a part of your life. You may and probably will have to make some adjustments in your lifestyle; the type and extent will depend upon your specific situation. Sometimes your symptoms will get worse, and you will be able to attribute it to the weather or your level of activity. At other times, it will get worse regardless of what you have or haven't done; sometimes it will just be beyond your control. Don't spend a lot of time worrying about what made you feel worse at the time. The important thing to keep in mind is that you need to learn what has become "normal" for you, acknowledging the reality of those limitations, without overcompensating. You need to become health conscious without focusing your entire life on your fibromyalgia. There will be times when you decide that the price you pay for doing something that brings you pleasure is justified. But, at this point, the first step in your treatment is realizing that fibromyalgia is going to change your life and deciding whether you will let its presence keep you from *living* with it.

The Basic Symptoms

Perhaps the strongest symptom in fibromyalgia is the presence of pain, pain that can be found all over the body. When the Criteria Committee for the American College of Rheumatology examined the records from 16 medical centers across the United States and Canada, they found that widespread pain was present in 97% of the cases diagnosed as fibromyalgia.

Widespread Pain

Widespread pain tends to occur along the skeleton, in the cervical (neck) area, chest, upper and lower back, shoulders, and hips. It has been described as aching, burning, radiating, spreading, gnawing, and shooting and is sometimes caused or aggravated by muscle spasms. Often it is hard to pinpoint the *exact* location of the pain, as it can be scattered.

The criteria set forth by the American College of Rheumatology specifies that the pain must be present in all four quadrants (left and right sides, above and below the waist). There is almost always lower back involvement. It is also necessary that pain be present for more than three months. An acute injury or ailment could be the cause of such pain, but once it has lasted more than three months, it becomes classified as chronic.

For many individuals, the pain begins in one spot and then moves to an overall pattern. One woman says, "I first began having pain in my neck and shoulders around 1968, which was diagnosed as 'tension'." Her symptoms have gradually increased so that now she feels pain in her lower back, thighs, hips, shoulders, and neck.

When I was serving in the U.S. Navy at Pensacola, Florida, I was required to participate in the regular physical fitness tests. The Navy WAVE officers wanted to make the exercises more interesting, so they brought in some of the Navy pilots' physical education instructors, who assigned exercises that placed major stress on my lower back. Everyone experienced sore muscles on the days following the exercises. My situation was more serious because my soreness didn't go away; instead, it got much worse; I had severe pain in my hips and lower back that kept me from taking anything but short, painful steps. It took four months in the hospital with physical therapy to relieve the pain. Through the next few years the primary location of my pain was in my lower back and hips.

With FM, people experience a general overall aching that is similar to the aches that accompany the flu. This aching is often present even when the sharper pain is absent. When asked where they hurt, many of those with FM reply, "All over."

Several studies have been conducted to determine the severity of fibromyalgia pain. As in other areas of research, these tests often contradict each other. The pain of fibromyalgia has been compared to that of both rheumatoid arthritis and osteoarthritis. One of the problems is that there is no one way to test the presence and severity of pain. It is subjective. The pain response can be affected by everything from the individual's ethnic and environmental background to his or her fatigue level.

Just as the degree of fibromyalgia pain is in question, so is the source of the pain. Extensive investigations of the muscles of people with FM have failed to turn up a physical cause for the pain. A few tests have found *microtrauma* (a microscopic lesion) to muscle tissue and possible shortage of blood flow to the muscles. But more research must be done.

For many people with fibromyalgia, just the acceptance of the pain and a clear diagnosis that transcends the "it's all in your head" theory are steps in the right direction. The lucky ones are those who have secured a positive diagnosis within a short time from the onset of symptoms.

The Tender Points

The second strongest symptom of fibromyalgia is the presence of tender points. Dr. Hugh Smythe first suggested that tender points be used as part of the diagnosis, suggesting that 12 of 14 such points be a positive sign. During the late 1970s and 1980s, researchers and doctors increased the number of tender-point locations to 75, using various percentages to indicate a positive diagnosis. There was no clear standard established until the Criteria Committee met in 1989.

Finally, in 1989, the Criteria Committee decided on 18 sites, located on both sides of the body and in areas above and below the waist. In the study conducted by the committee, the presence of the tender points was the most powerful indicator separating those with fibromyalgia from those without. In the control, or normal, group, subjects felt a slight tenderness but no actual pain when pressure was applied to a tender point.

But when that same amount of pressure was applied to a tender point on a person with fibromyalgia, the examiner got an intense pain response, with the person often pulling away. In early studies, doctors looked for that jump reflex.

There are several reasons that these tender points are important, particularly to a person with FM. Because of the early tendency to attribute the pain and fatigue to psychological problems, the discovery of these sites of pain was a great relief. The reason that the medical community endorses the tender-point theory is that the person being tested has no knowledge of such points and, therefore, cannot not fake that pain.

Tender points are in specific locations. They are situated at the bony insertions of tendons or at a muscle-bone interface. If the examiner is off even centimeters from the indicated spot, the response is not the same.

In addition to relying on the presence of the tender points to disprove a mental illness diagnosis, now we also know that psychogenic rheumatism, which is a manifestation of a psychological problem, produces erratic and bizarre symptoms, none of which can be reproduced by an examiner.

Because it was often difficult to apply a consistent amount of pressure, many doctors began to use a simple spring-loaded gauge, called a *dolorimeter,* which enabled them to be precise in measuring the amount of pressure they applied. The committee determined that the pressure must be applied with an approximate force of 4 kg. And, of course, they also determined that at least 11 of the 18 points should register positive for the diagnosis of FM. The 18 sites are the following:

- Sites 1 and 2—Occiput: bilateral, at the suboccipital muscle insertions
- Sites 3 and 4—Low cervical: bilateral, at the anterior aspects of the intertransverse spaces at C5–C7
- Sites 5 and 6—Trapezius: bilateral, at the midpoint of the upper border
- Sites 7 and 8—Supraspinatus: bilateral, at origins, above the spine of the scapula near the medial border
- Sites 9 and 10—Second rib: bilateral, at the second costochondral junctions, just lateral to the junctions on upper surfaces
- Sites 11 and 12—Lateral epicondyle: bilateral, 2 cm distal to the epicondyles
- Sites 13 and 14—Gluteal: bilateral, in upper quadrants of buttocks in anterior fold of muscle

- Sits 15 and 16—Greater trochanter: bilateral, posterior to the trochanteric prominence
- Sits 17 and 18—Knee: bilateral, at the medial fat pad proximal to the joint line

Characteristics of Fibromyalgia

"I've had a total reversal of lifestyle. I was working full-time at a challenging, good-paying job. Recreational activities included hiking in the mountains, swimming 120 laps a day in a 25-meter pool, aerobic exercises, and dancercize."

FATIGUE

Fatigue presents almost as much of a problem for the person with FM as the pain does. Quite often it is possible to concentrate on something else, to take your mind off the pain much of the time, but fatigue can leave you without the ability even to concentrate.

As mentioned once before, the effects of fibromyalgia vary from person to person; some people are only aware of a tired feeling after exertion. These people may need no more than a short nap in the afternoon to continue their normal activities. For others, however, even minor exertion produces extreme fatigue, requiring them to rest often.

People with FM often find that short periods of exertion require much longer periods of rest to recuperate. One person says that for a half hour of exertion, she needs at least a full hour to recover. As a result, it takes much longer to complete tasks because frequent rest stops are necessary. One of the most common complaints from people with FM is that they are no longer able to do even normal daily tasks. They worry about returning to full- or even part-time work when they need help with the basic activities necessary to maintain day-to-day life.

Sometimes shortness of breath occurs, and some physicians have speculated that the fatigue, and hence the shortness of breath, is related to being out of shape or "deconditioned." Dr. Moldofsky's original study on sleep deprivation supports this possibility because it reproduced fibrositis symptoms in all of his subjects but two. Those two were in excellent physical condition, as they were on a college track team and ran seven miles a day.

Since that study, a number of studies have looked at the role muscles and

Tender Point Sites

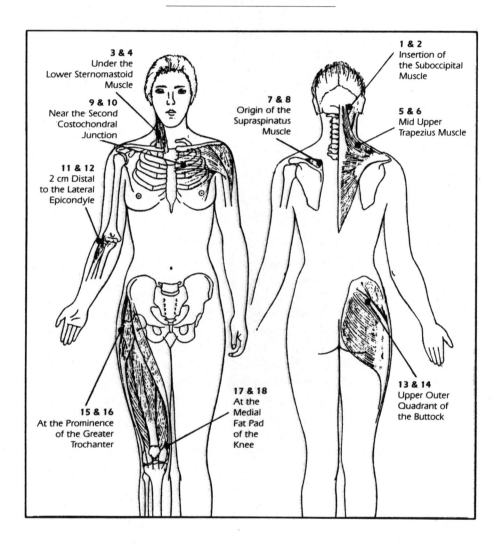

aerobic fitness play in FM. Some research indicates that if a person with FM works to become aerobically fit, the FM symptoms will ease. For some, this is true. For others, pain remains even when they engage in regular aerobic exercise. And in the case of still others, even mild exercise brings severe pain.

Up to this point, nothing decisive has been found to answer the questions of why muscle pain and exhaustion occur, but current studies are examining the effects of muscle metabolism, regional blood flow, and respiratory gas exchanges on FM. One important link that has been evident since the late 1970s, although its role in causing FM has yet to be determined, is the nonrestorative sleep pattern seen in a majority of those with FM.

NONRESTORATIVE SLEEP

If the focus of the question is on the ability to fall asleep and stay asleep, many people with FM say they don't have a problem, when questioned about their sleep habits. However, if asked how they feel when they get up in the morning, most say they feel terrible.

No matter how many hours of sleep they get, almost 100% of people with FM awake unrested. Dr. Moldofsky has been studying the sleep problems associated with FM for a number of years. His research has demonstrated an intrusion of *alpha*, or waking, brain waves, into the *delta* waves of stage-four, or non-rapid-eye-movement (non-REM), sleep (the stage of sleep that restores the body's energy). This is called alpha-delta sleep. When Dr. Moldofsky continually interrupted the stage-four sleep of healthy subjects, they developed the fatigue, musculoskeletal pain, and tender points typical of fibromyalgia.

However, new studies have found that the intrusion of alpha waves not only is present in the delta, or deep, sleep but also can occur in stages one and two and even, though rarely, in the REM, or rapid-eye-movement, sleep. The new term for this, according to Dr. Moldofsky, is alpha EEG (electroencephalographic) NREM sleep anomaly. Other studies have shown that while normal controls or those with chronic insomnia (dysthymia) may have approximately 25% of their NREM-stage sleep interrupted with alpha wave intrusions, those with fibromyalgia have about 60% of their NREM-stage sleep interrupted. Interestingly, there are individuals who have the alpha-delta intrusion but do not have the symptoms of fibromyalgia. This has caused doctors and researchers to wonder if there are certain individuals who may be predisposed to the condition and eventually develop FM once it is triggered by an accident, illness, or a stress-related state of crisis. This idea is one that is still being explored.

These intrusions of alpha waves into the delta, or deep, sleep waves have been compared to an internal arousal mechanism that kicks in on a regular basis. It may be this mechanism that pulls sleepers out of their restorative sleep, leaving them tired and in pain. The level of pain seems to be directly correlated to the length of time that delta-wave sleep was disrupted.

When trying to determine what causes the alpha EEG NREM sleep anomaly, a number of factors have been considered, including psychological stress, environmental events, primary sleep and physiology disorders, and painful joint problems.

FACTORS IMPORTANT IN SUSPECTING SLEEP DISTURBANCE

- Difficulty in initiating sleep
- Difficulty maintaining sleep
- Fatigue on awakening
- Pain and stiffness on awakening
- Excessive sleepiness or napping during the day or evening
- Vigorous exercise in the evening
- Excessive fluids after dinner
- Excessive caffeine
- Excessive alcohol
- Excessive heavy or spicy foods in the evening
- Watching television before bedtime
- Eating before bedtime
- Nocturia (the need to urinate at night)
- Excessive noise
- Uncomfortable mattress
- Poorly controlled temperature
- Sleep medication
- Periodic leg movements
- Restlessness
- Snoring
- Pets in the bedroom or on the bed
- Excessive stress

Courtesy of Dr. P. Kahler Hench. Reprinted with permission from *Rheumatic Disease Clinics of North America.*

Studies have been conducted on all of the suspected sleep disturbances but as with all other aspects of FM, more need to be done. People who experienced a noninjury automobile or industrial accident and developed sleep disturbances and musculoskeletal pain have been compared to people who had no known cause for their fibrositis symptoms. Those who had an accident or experienced domestic problems from which they could not extricate themselves showed much stronger sleep anomalies.

Problems with the sleep environment have also been proven to cause disruption. Many people with fibromyalgia have indicated a sensitivity to noise that may explain their sleep problems. Studies conducted near airports have shown that residents report sleep problems, fatigue, rheumatic pain, and emotional distress. Other studies suggest that the wrong bedroom temperature, the presence of young children, having pets in the room or on the bed, and even sharing the bed with someone who snores may disrupt sleep.

FACTORS PHYSICIANS HAVE FOUND TO HAVE A NEGATIVE EFFECT ON THE SLEEP OF PEOPLE WITH FIBROMYALGIA

- Intrusion of alpha waves into stage-four delta-wave sleep
- Bruxism (grinding teeth during sleep)
- Nocturnal myoclonus (periodic leg movements)
- Sleep apnea (temporary cessation of breathing)
- Narcolepsy (extreme tendency to fall asleep whenever in a quiet environment)
- Nocturnal hypnogenic myoclonus (nighttime hypnotic state with periodic leg movements)
- Arthritic pain (rheumatoid arthritis and osteoarthritis)
- Stress
- Symptoms of concomitant illness
- Nocturia (passage of urine at night)
- Pain

Courtesy of Dr. P. Kahler Hench. Reprinted with permission from *Rheumatic Disease Clinics of North America*.

One study, on people who have obstructive *sleep apnea* (obstructed and irregular breathing during sleep) and sleep-related periodic involuntary leg movements showed a worsening of fibromyalgia symptoms. However, they also reported daytime somnolence, which has not been tied to FM. Those in the study that did have sleep-related leg movements tended to be women and tended to have more musculoskeletal pain, fatigue, and sleep-stage changes.

Studies involving people with rheumatoid arthritis and osteoarthritis have shown them to have more symptoms with alpha EEG NREM sleep anomalies. The question seems to be which caused the problems? Did the pain of the arthritis affect the sleep of the individual, or did the sleep disturbance increase the pain, morning stiffness, and fatigue usually associated with these conditions?

Because fibromyalgia is considered a syndrome (research has not been able to prove it is a disease) treatment at this time deals with managing the symptoms. We will look more extensively at the treatment of the sleep disturbance later, but generally, small doses of tricyclic antidepressant medications such as Elavil, Endep, and Flexeril are given to improve sleep quality. Elavil and Endep (both brand names for *amitriptyline*) and Flexeril *(cyclobenzaprine HCl)* are given in small doses at bedtime and have shown some improvement. The doses are much less than what would be prescribed to treat depression.

MORNING STIFFNESS

"It takes me nearly an hour to work out my stiffness when I get up in the morning."

The morning stiffness of fibromyalgia has been compared to that experienced by people who have rheumatoid arthritis, although there is no real explanation for it. One theory suggests a physiological problem may be the answer. As Dr. Xavier Caro explained in the *Fibromyalgia Network Newsletter* (April 1990), "It is due to the accumulation of tissue fluids and mediated, at least in part, by a lesion of increased vascular permeability. In other words, proteins and other substances are able to leak through the blood vessel wall barriers (due to these small vascular lesions) and accumulate in the tissue areas where they are not supposed to be."

Some people report a staggering or stumbling walk when they first get out of bed in the morning. This seems to be caused by the stiffness and eases as the person walks around. During the day, keeping a limb or hand in one position or sitting for a prolonged time may cause the stiffness to return.

Common Conditions of Fibromyalgia

In addition to the common features identified by Dr. Wolfe, there are other conditions that often appear in people with fibromyalgia. These conditions include psychological abnormalities such as depression, irritable bowel syndrome, headaches, *paresthesias* (abnormal sensations without objective cause, such as numbness, prickling, tingling, and heightened sensitivity), and subjective swelling (a swelling sensation). There is also a small percentage of people who have some functional disability.

Psychological Abnormalities

"JUST BITCHY WOMEN WHOSE SYMPTOMS ARE ALL IN THEIR HEAD"

In 1987, when I first began to research fibromyalgia, a member of the Arthritis Foundation shared this quote with me and told me that the medical community had regarded the syndrome this way in the past. Many of those with FM are still fighting that tag.

Quite a bit has been written regarding the psychological state of those with FM. In the past, belief in the psychological diagnosis for FM has been compounded by the use of certain psychological tests. But the opinion among researchers currently working on FM appears to be changing. Dr. Frederick Wolfe felt that the *Minnesota Multiphasic Personality Inventory* (MMPI), a psychological test that helps determine psychological problems such as depression, was only one tool and perhaps an imperfect one for assessing the existence of significant psychological problems. Dr. Hugh Smythe also felt that the MMPI was an inadequate instrument for the evaluation of the psychologic status of rheumatic disease patients.

It was a team of researchers at Oregon Health Sciences University in Portland, Oregon, whose results were published in *Arthritis and Rheumatism* in 1985, who produced some of the most important findings on this aspect of FM. They were the first researchers to choose patients from a regular medical clinic rather than from a rheumatology practice. This is important because Sharon Clark, R.N., Ph.D., and two doctors who have since led much of the research on FM, Dr. Robert Bennett and Dr. Stephen Campbell, were able to show that there was no difference in the psychological states of the control subjects and the FM patients. After considering their results, the Oregon research team declared, "A number of other findings, including the response of the pain to weather fronts, the marked stiffness reminiscent of other rheumatic diseases, the consistent location of the fibrositic tender points, the occasional finding of palpable nodules with electromyographic and histologic abnormalities, and the disturbance of sleep all suggest a peripheral or, at least, non-psychogenic component of the disease."

Clark's team also felt that the psychological abnormalities the FM sufferers experienced were the result of psychological components that did register and were caused by the chronic or severe pain and disability as well as their anxiety about the nature or actual existence of a disease. They also found that the patients in previous studies had been selected either while hospitalized or while being seen by rheumatologists and therefore were those who had more severe physical symptoms.

Several more studies were done over the next few years, and again the results pointed to problems with the testing. The major difficulty seemed to be reflected in five disease-related statements that were consistently more common in the profiles of rheumatoid arthritis patients as well as those with FM. Those five statements were:

1. I wake up fresh and rested most mornings.
2. I am about as able to work as I ever was.
3. I seldom worry about my health.
4. I am in just as good physical health as most of my friends.
5. I have little or no pain.

Almost anyone with fibromyalgia would respond to these statements negatively. Response patterns to the five disease-related items are associated with the severity of pain, determined by health assessment questionnaire (HAQ) scores and grip-strength measures, as well as the presence of disease. The final recommendation was that new criteria were needed to validate using the MMPI as a clinical tool for recognizing hypochondriasis, depression, and hysteria in anyone who has chronic pain.

Other studies showed there *was* a relationship between fibromyalgia and *major affective* (mood) disorder as well as a familial predisposition to both depression and fibromyalgia. The general consensus is that both fibromyalgia and its associated *psychopathology* (mental illness) are caused by a common but unknown abnormality. There is also the possibility that several other medical and psychiatric disorders that share common *pathophysiologic* (body functions that are no longer functioning normally) features are linked. These include conditions that are often seen in those with FM, including irritable bowel syndrome, migraine headaches, major depression, and a panic disorder.

Dr. Harold Merskey, London Psychiatric Hospital, London, Ontario, evaluated many of the present methods used to test for psychological problems and found some of the same problems noted by Smythe, Wolfe, and others. Dr. Merskey says these tests show that psychiatric illnesses may affect as few as 30% of patients with FM in some series of studies. He cited selection bias and the fact that many of the resulting psychological disturbances would be considered secondary to pain and disability and could even be attributed to insomnia and anxiety.

Dr. Don Goldenberg, at Boston University School of Medicine, has become one of the leaders in research on fibromyalgia. He was primarily responsible for the 1990 conference on FM and chronic fatigue syndrome held in California. Author of a number of articles on the psychological effects of fibromyalgia, Dr. Goldenberg emphatically says:

Recent studies do not support the notion that fibromyalgia is a psychiatric disorder. There is no evidence that fibromyalgia is a hysterical or a somatization disorder. There may be a significant association of fibromyalgia and depression or depressive symptoms but the meaning and mechanism of this association is not yet known.

Dr. Muhammad B. Yunus and others in the Department of Medicine at the University of Illinois at Peoria, studied the relationship of clinical features and psychological status in fibromyalgia. They found that the MMPI was a valid test for assessing the psychological status of those with fibromyalgia.

Based on the concept that those with FM should be subgrouped into three psychological categories including normal profile, typical chronic pain profile, and psychological disturbance profile, the group compared the clinical features of FM (tender points, fatigue, and poor sleep) and other symptoms such as severe pain, swelling, and paresthesia. The results showed no direct correlation between the central features of fibromyalgia and the psychological status as shown by the MMPI results or with individual MMPI scales. The one feature of pain severity may be influenced by psychological factors. The researchers concluded, "It appears that fibromyalgia is a multidimensional syndrome in which

CONCLUSIONS FROM PRIOR STUDIES OF PSYCHOLOGICAL ASSOCIATIONS WITH FIBROMYALGIA AND SUGGESTIONS FOR FUTURE STUDIES

- The majority (65% to 80%) of people with fibromyalgia do not have an active psychiatric disorder. A subgroup of people may have significant active psychopathology. This group should be better delineated and evaluated.
- There may be a greater prevalence of depression in people with fibromyalgia compared with rheumatoid arthritis, although some studies have not found such differences. Most studies do find a greater prevalence of symptoms of depression in those with rheumatoid arthritis, fibromyalgia, or any chronic medical illness than in people with other medical problems.
- There may also be a greater lifetime history and family history of depression in people with fibromyalgia compared to rheumatoid arthritis patients and controls. These may indicate some psychological link that should be investigated.
- Psychological tests such as the MMPI and even a structured interview technique such as the diagnostic interview schedule (DIS) do not adequately work for chronic pain and associated medical conditions. Such tests need to be modified for use in medical patients and then validated in various chronic pain disorders. Previous reports of psychopathology in people with fibromyalgia may have reflected disease activity reporting.
- Future studies should select psychiatric tests that are less affected by chronic pain. The effect of medications on symptoms of pain should be distinguished from their effect on mood and psyche. Antidepressant doses as well as smaller doses of antidepressants could then be better evaluated regarding their effect on fibromyalgia. The psychiatric state of a person should be known, either by prospective studies, or by structured historical interview data.

Courtesy of Dr. Don L. Goldenberg. Reprinted with permission from *Rheumatic Disease Clinics of North America*.

psychological factors may influence the degree of pain and perhaps the referral pattern [to rheumatology clinics]."

It is encouraging to be assured that the symptoms are *not* mentally induced. It provides hope that someday not only will someone discover the cause of the pain and fatigue but that an effective treatment will also be found. Most of us recognize that stress plays a part in FM. We can accept that both emotional and physical stress exacerbate the symptoms, knowing that there is, somewhere, a physical cause for our problems.

Irritable Bowel Syndrome

Many links have been indicated between fibromyalgia and irritable bowel syndrome (IBS) in a collection of medical journals. But only recently have studies become directed to the relationship between the two and the fact that they may have more in common than previously believed.

Irritable bowel syndrome usually occurs when a person experiences abdominal pain that is related to defecation, alternating diarrhea and constipation, abdominal distension, gas, and excessive mucus in the stool. Even though IBS affects nearly 30% of the patients who seek medical help for gastrointestinal symptoms, many who have such symptoms never seek medical attention for them. Dr. Wolfe includes IBS in the common features that affect more than 25% of people who have FM.

Dr. George Triadafilopoulos, Dr. Robert Simms, and Dr. Goldenberg, from the Section of Gastroenterology and Arthritis and the Evans Memorial Department of Clinical Research at the University Hospital in Boston studied 123 individuals with fibromyalgia for the presence of either irritable bowel syndrome or bowel dysfunction and reported their findings in the January, 1991 issue of *Digestive Diseases and Science.* Results showed a large number of people with FM felt that they had altered bowel functions. One of the most interesting aspects of the study showed that the subjects' gastrointestinal symptoms were exacerbated when their fibromyalgia symptoms flared up, as well as when they experienced stress. This worsening of both conditions has also been reported by Dr. Muhammad Yunus and his associates at the University of Illinois.

Dr. Triadafilopoulos and associates concluded that their research "supports the notion that fibromyalgia is not a disorder with impact solely on the musculoskeletal system and that other psychophysiological factors [dealing with both the body and the mind] may be involved."

Like fibromyalgia, irritable bowel syndrome has no organic base and is often affected by psychological stress as well as diet. Sleep disturbance has been reported in up to 30% of IBS patients in at least one study. One theory suggests that a generalized, genetically determined disorder affects smooth muscle, which would tie in other conditions often associated with both FM and IBS, such as dysmenorrhea (painful menstrual cramps) and migraines. The common link lies in the smooth muscle which has a genetic tendency to behave abnormally.

Dr. D. Veale, at Beumont Hospital in Dublin, Ireland, questions the possibility of that tendency to also affect striated muscle (the type of muscle found to be painful in FM) and asserts, "Factors such as diet, physical exercise, poor sleep pattern and psychological stress may determine which symptom complex predominates." He suggests that a high-fiber diet study be conducted with FM individuals and that a strong exercise program, complimented by low doses of the tricyclic antidepressants, be tested on those with IBS.

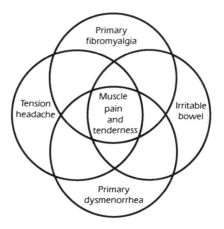

PRIMARY FIBROMYALGIA, IRRITABLE BOWEL, PRIMARY DYSMENORRHEA AND TENSION HEADACHE SHARE MANY COMMON FEATURES, INCLUDING MUSCLE PAIN AND TENDERNESS.

Courtesy of Dr. Muhammad B. Yunus.
Reprinted with permission from the *Journal of Rheumatology*.

Headaches and More

Tension and migraine headaches have been consistently noted in some people with fibromyalgia throughout the last 15 years of research on FM. Many report chronic diffuse and bilateral headaches that are affected by emotional stress and are not caused by another condition. Although there has been no research solely on the prevalence of such headaches, a number of studies have included discussion on the presence of them. In the May, 1987 issue of the *Journal of the American Medical Association,* Dr. Goldenberg, compared three previous studies on fibromyalgia with his own. Bothersome headaches were present in 55% of the subjects in Dr. Goldenberg's study, in 44% of the subjects in one conducted by Dr. Muhammad Yunus, in 56% of the subjects in Dr. Frederick Wolfe's and Mary Ann Cathey's study, and in 55% of the subjects in one conducted by Dr. Stephen Campbell and his associates.

But there are also other symptoms that are often found to accompany fibromyalgia. Many people report subjective swelling, particularly in their hands and fingers; however, there is no objective basis for evaluating the swelling. Paresthesia is also very common. No organic reason for these sensations has been found, yet they are reported by many people with FM.

Reports of increased sensitivity to many factors such as cold, noise, some foods and drugs have also been made. Raynaud's syndrome or a Raynaud-like syndrome is reported to occur in the hands and feet of 30% to 40% of those with FM. Dr. Bennett believes the occurrence of the Raynaud-like condition is not caused by a disease of the blood vessels. It is common to women, usually starting after they have begun to menstruate, and may be linked to hormones.

There is the possibility that fibromyalgia also may have a hormonal link, since it predominantly affects women, and many are affected around the time of menopause. Some women find that they have worse pain during the first days of their periods and that it often radiates to the lower back and upper thighs. There may be a link between painful menstrual cramps and FM, but nothing has been proven yet.

Sicca symptoms have also been found in those with FM. This is a condition that leaves the mouth, eyes, and other areas of mucous membranes dry. To confirm the condition, a *Schirmer test* is conducted. For this test, a standard filter paper is placed inside the lower eyelid of each anesthetized eye for five minutes. (It should be noted that people who are taking antidepressants, Flexeril, or certain other drugs may experience a dry mouth and nose as a side effect; there are a number of other conditions that also include such symptoms.)

As previously mentioned, people with FM experience shortness of breath. Five doctors from the Department of Rehabilitation Medicine and the Department of Clinical Physiology at Sahlgren's University Hospital in Gothenburg, Sweden, conducted studies on shortness of breath, or *dyspnea* (labored or difficult breathing). They concluded that such shortness of breath is common in people who have FM and may be due in part to diaphragmatic muscular insufficiency and the physical inactivity present in many with FM.

There is a theory that chronic fatigue syndrome and fibromyalgia may be two sides of a coin. Dr. Goldenberg is the leading proponent of this theory. He has found similarities of symptoms in the two groups and asserts that there may be a potential role for virally induced immune dysfunction for both FM and chronic fatigue syndrome (CFS). In March, 1990 Dr. Goldenberg reported that these similarities were being investigated and said "Studies include the roles that may be played by specific viruses, possible immune-mediated events, similar types of sleep disturbances, the frequency and effect of depression, and other neuropsychiatric symptoms and histochemical evaluations (lab work) of muscle hypoxia (lack of oxygen to the muscles)."

Often people with FM find it difficult to determine whether a symptom is caused by FM or a totally different health problem. Too often they feel like the little boy who cried wolf; they decide that the symptom must be an aspect of fibromyalgia and since there is only so much that can be done, they ignore it. Only your health professional can tell you for sure. If you have had a symptom for some time and your doctor tells you not to worry, use your common sense. How bad is it? Is it sharp or dull pain? Is it constant or intermittent? Is it possible it could be something else entirely?

Without running to a doctor for every new symptom, you must learn to evaluate such symptoms carefully. It may or may not be FM. Just because you have fibromyalgia doesn't mean that you can't develop some other serious health problem. If there is any question in your mind at all, consult your doctor.

Looking into Treatment

If you believe that you have fibromyalgia, you need to obtain a firm diagnosis. That means finding a doctor who knows something about fibromyalgia and is willing to work with you. It might seem as if the two requirements would be the same, but, unfortunately, there are some doctors who know about FM and choose not to treat it or take on new cases. If that is the case, then you are better off continuing your search. Treating FM can be frustrating and time-consuming for the doctor as well as for the person with FM.

One person wrote, "I struggled so long to overcome pain. My family M.D. tried—he tried his best to treat my 'rheumatoid arthritis'. But he got tired of me, as I grew more demanding for relief. I was very hurt by his diagnosis of 'chronic pain'—somehow to me, 'chronic pain' meant *I* was at fault. But now I know that because all the medications were useless, my doctor himself was feeling frustrated. He realized it couldn't be arthritis or bursitis, but he didn't know what it was, so to meet the insurance company's demand for diagnosis, he wrote 'chronic pain'."

Too many times doctors do not want to admit to you, and perhaps to themselves, that they don't know what is wrong and don't know how to treat it. Even in this day, when medicine has progressed so far, there are a lot of health problems that remain a mystery. Dr. Jay Goldstein has written a book, titled *Could Your Doctor Be Wrong?* (Pharos Books), for people whose symptoms and health problems don't fit into the cookbook that physicians are taught in medical school. I highly recommend it to those who have felt they never quite fit into the nice, neat box of known illnesses.

So how do you find the doctor who knows something about fibromyalgia and is willing to work with you? There are a number of ways to locate such a doctor. First, contact your local Arthritis Foundation chapter (see the appendix for a list of chapters in the United States). They usually provide a list of rheumatologists in their areas.

If you live near a medical university, contact their rheumatology clinic.

There are several advantages in choosing medical professionals affiliated with a medical university. They may be conducting studies you could take part in. Whenever possible, those with FM should participate in research. After all, the more research that is conducted, the better chance researchers have of finding the causes and treatments for FM.

Another advantage of choosing a clinic affiliated with a university is the possibility of reduced fees. This is not always the case, but if you have no insurance and money is a consideration, you might check into it.

When a medical university has clinical facilities, medical students observe and work in the clinics under a staff physician's supervision. I have always welcomed their presence during my appointments with the doctor; this gives them the opportunity to learn more about fibromyalgia. If you are uncomfortable with the idea of medical students participating in your care, then a medical university clinic is not for you.

If there is no such facility available in your area, look for a fibromyalgia support group. (See the appendix for a list of groups, but keep in mind that there are undoubtedly many others.) Call your local hospital or newspaper to find out if there is a group meeting near you. Very often support groups have a list of doctors who treat FM. While many groups are hesitant to openly endorse or denounce the doctors in their areas, they usually know which doctors are knowledgeable about FM and which ones will work with you.

If there is no Arthritis Foundation chapter, no support group, and no list of such doctors in your area, consider interviewing rheumatologists or family practitioners. This concept is still so new that many people feel uncomfortable taking this approach. You should not feel this way. You must be an active partner in your health care. No doctor is going to have a pill that will cure your FM. Even with medicine, physical therapy, and other forms of treatment, you may still have bothersome symptoms. There is only so much that medical personnel can do—the rest is up to you. After all, you live in your body 24 hours a day. You are the primary factor in your treatment. Therefore, you want to be able to work with the doctor to get the best results from whatever treatment the two of you choose.

Once you have found a doctor who agrees to treat you and who is experienced in treating FM, you should be able to develop a program that is tailored for you and your symptoms. Everyone is different and each person's case is different. Don't compare yourself with someone who has it "better" or "worse" than you. This isn't a contest. This month you might need intensive physical therapy, but two months from now you might need to increase your medication or you might need someone who can understand the anger and depression you experience when your body refuses to let you do something you want to do. Once you arrive at this understanding, you will have begun living "the first day of the rest of your life."

The severity of your symptoms and the needs of your lifestyle will determine the means of treatment. It may be necessary to try a number of drugs,
modes of treatment, or combinations thereof to find what works best. Don't
expect a miracle cure. There isn't one. Mild medication enables some people to
sleep better and they see an improvement almost immediately. For others, it
may take a period of hospitalization to break the pain cycle. Although many of
those seeking a diagnosis for fibromyalgia have spent a lot of time in hospitals
during their search, once they get a diagnosis, their frequency of hospitalization
decreases dramatically.

If you already have a doctor who is treating your fibromyalgia, ask yourself
if you are happy with your relationship. Of the people I have surveyed, about
25% were not satisfied with their doctors. Many of them felt they knew more
about FM than their doctors did or indicated their doctors never took the time
to talk with them.

However, it is encouraging that almost 50% of the group felt their doctors
were knowledgeable and caring. Their doctors took the time to sit down and
talk with them about fibromyalgia, its impact, and its treatment. This is a great
improvement from the time when a "good patient" was one who asked no
questions and left everything to the doctor. This style of doctoring has almost
disappeared, as both doctors and patients realize that the physician is human
and also has good and bad days. You can help facilitate excellent care by carefully writing down any questions you may have or anything that you do not
understand. This helps both of you address what you need to know during the
office visit.

In the research literature on FM, the authors consistently encourage doctors to take the time to discuss FM with their patients and to reassure them. This
assurance and your active involvement provide the foundation for living with
FM.

Whatever other specialists your doctor involves, you will often find that it
takes all of them to produce some advances in your treatment. Treatment must
be interdisciplinary. We are made up of body, mind, and spirit, and modern
medicine is finally recognizing that they are so intricately intertwined that it is
impossible to separate them. We will look at the treatments that affect the body
first, then the mind, and lastly, the spirit.

WHAT YOUR DOCTOR MAY DO AND SAY

1. Reassure you that the syndrome is a real medical entity but
   is not progressive, crippling, or life threatening.
2. Point out that prospects for medical cure are only moderate.

3. Identify and treat concomitant painful conditions, psychological disturbances, or other factors that may exacerbate or contribute to symptoms.
4. Suggest positive environmental changes.
5. Encourage you to:
   - take an active role in the management of the disease;
   - correct stresses to the cervical and lumbar spine by the use of neck-support pillows during sleep and abdominal exercises to strengthen muscular support of the back;
   - begin a gradually progressive program of aerobic exercise to improve the level of muscular fitness and sense of well-being;
   - remain physically and socially active;
   - identify and eliminate stresses or environmental disturbances that may exacerbate sleep disturbance and symptoms;
   - avoid using the diagnosis for secondary gain, such as avoidance of unwelcome tasks;
   - avoid overdependence on medical personnel or resources.
6. Prescribe low doses of tricyclic medications to improve sleep quality.
7. Prescribe simple analgesics, such as acetaminophen, as needed.

Courtesy of Dr. Robert M. Bennett. Reprinted with permission from *Patient Care*.

Okay, now you have a doctor and you know something about FM—it's time to set up your game plan. What kind of drugs are available? What about physical therapy? How can you control your pain? Just how effective is a particular mode of treatment? Remember, you are striving to break the pain cycle, to obtain whatever relief the medical personnel can give you, and then to make some changes in your lifestyle that will extend the relief.

Let's start with the drugs.

Medication

Because the cause of fibromyalgia is unknown, treatment must concentrate on alleviating the symptoms. Those symptoms include the widespread pain, muscle spasms, and sleep disturbance. Sometimes by treating the sleep disturbance, the pain and the muscle spasms can be relieved. Different drugs from several categories are prescribed for those with FM.

ANALGESICS

The use of such simple *analgesics* as aspirin or *acetaminophen* can relieve most of the pain for some people and enable them to sleep more comfortably. For six years I was able to control my pain with these over-the-counter drugs. Several of the people I surveyed have indicated that these are all they need except in special situations. Some take Ecotrin or another coated aspirin to prevent stomach upset.

NONSTEROIDAL ANTI-INFLAMMATORY DRUGS

Because FM is a chronic syndrome, pain relief from drugs must be handled carefully. An addiction to painkillers will only complicate matters. Therefore, initial relief is sought from nonsteroidal anti-inflammatory drugs. There is no inflammation as in other rheumatic conditions, so these drugs are looked to more for their painkilling effects than for their anti-inflammatory action. Just as in other rheumatic conditions, they are often prescribed on a continuous basis in an attempt to establish a certain level of the drug in the bloodstream.

Generally, the range of nonsteroidal anti-inflammatory drugs is tried in an attempt to find one that works best for the individual. The major problem with these drugs is not potential addiction but the damage they can do to the stomach. Unfortunately, few drugs have no side effects, so we end up treating the major health problem (pain) and then have to treat the side effect of the painkiller (irritated stomach).

TRICYCLIC MEDICATIONS

Because sleep disturbance has been indicated as the source of increased pain and fatigue, medications that improve sleep are used. Initially, Dr. Harvey Moldofsky's sleep studies seemed to indicate that the sleep disturbances were tied into the fatigue and chronic pain. This idea led to seeking drugs that would increase the stage-four, or non-rapid-eye-movement restorative sleep.

Tricyclic antidepressants such as amitriptyline (Elavil or Endep) have been shown to have an impact on the central and peripheral nervous system. And early studies demonstrated a positive response to amitriptyline in people with FM on a short-term basis. However, follow-ups on many of those who took part in the study found that positive response was lost over a period of time, and that the symptoms remained fairly stable, returning to their original level.

Tricyclics can reduce the alpha-wave intrusions into stage-four NREM sleep, block the re-uptake of *norepinephrine* and *serotonin* (chemicals that help transmit pain signals), and increase endorphin stimulation levels.

The dosage used in the treatment of fibromyalgia is far lower than that normally given for depression. Quite often, when a physician suggests the use of a tricyclic antidepressant, the person with FM is quick to conclude that the doctor believes the problem is psychological. Dosage for chronic pain is generally no more than 10 mg to 40 mg per day, while that for depression can be as high as 150 mg to 200 mg per day.

Because of the nature of the symptoms of FM, it is hard to prove a drug's contribution to improvement. A study conducted at the University of Alberta by Dr. Roger Scudds and Dr. Glenn McCain, who is from the University of Western Ontario, sought improvements in "outcome measures of pain, tender point sensitivity and patient assessment of well-being." Their results showed improvement in overall myalgia as well as pain threshold and tolerance. The overall myalgia improvement came after the active treatment period, when the tender points became less responsive to pressure.

Tricyclic antidepressants remain the top medicines of choice for lack of better drugs.

MUSCLE RELAXANTS

Cyclobenzaprine (Flexeril) is another member of the tricyclic medicines, but it is primarily a muscle relaxer. It may affect the central nervous system as well as peripheral actions. Dr. Robert Bennett and others conducted a trial study comparing cyclobenzaprine and a placebo on 120 patients with fibromyalgia. The results showed improvement in the quality of sleep, a decrease in pain severity and level of fatigue, but showed no improvement in morning stiffness.

Other muscle relaxers sometimes prescribed are *methocarbamol* (Robaxin), *chlorozoxazone* (Paraflex), *chloroxazone* Parafon Forte, and *carisoprodol* (Soma).

BENZODIAZEPINES

Benzodiazepines are anti-anxiety drugs that have been helpful in reducing muscle spasms, pain, and sleep disturbance. *Alprazolam* (Xanax) is perhaps the one used most commonly and has been studied in combination with *ibuprofen*, producing improvements for some people with FM.

While all these drugs provide some relief for some people with fibromyalgia, none totally relieves all symptoms. Yet you shouldn't be pessimistic when starting out. Be willing to give your doctor and these drugs a try. You may end up like the 54-year-old teacher who was diagnosed in 1990 with FM and who has obtained relief with piroxicam. She says that her activities are not limited at the present time and that Feldene has almost completely relieved all her pain.

One more word about drugs. Learn as much as you can about this aspect of FM as well as all the others. Know what drugs your doctor has prescribed for you, how to take them, and what their side effects are. Make a point of telling each of your doctors, if you have more than one, what other medications you are taking. Often drug combinations will create serious side effects. If you don't tell your cardiologist what your rheumatologist has prescribed for you, and vice versa, you may experience serious problems.

Buy one of the excellent guides to prescription and over-the-counter drugs and keep it handy. If you can't read your doctor's prescription, make sure the pharmacy writes the generic or brand name of the drug on your bottle as well as clear instructions for taking the medicine.

Options for
Nondrug Treatment

For many people, nondrug treatment, such as physical therapy and osteopathic manipulation, is more likely to improve their condition than treatment with medication. Explore the nondrug treatments that are available to you. Although people with FM commonly get different results from the same methods of treatment, nondrug treatments usually produce positive results for most people.

Physical Therapy

Physical therapy for people with FM includes both passive and active modes. The main objective of physical therapy is to ease muscle spasms through relaxation, thereby easing pain. The second objective is to help you learn normal neuromuscular functioning. Physical therapy is done on either an inpatient or an outpatient basis. Hospitalization is usually necessary only when the pain is so severe that a combination of physical therapy and bed rest is required to break the pain-spasm-pain cycle, but most of the time it can be done on an outpatient basis.

Although new advances are being made daily in the study of pain, the chronic pain of fibromyalgia has proven difficult to understand. As mentioned earlier, no one is sure if the "end organ" in FM is the muscle or the central nervous system. Most physical therapy is directed toward the muscles to relieve the spasms. We will look at methods of treatment directed at the central nervous system later.

Relaxing the muscles begins with the application of either heat or cold. This usually involves the use of hot packs or cold packs applied to the painful areas. Many people feel better after the hot packs are applied, while others cannot tolerate the heat. That is not because the heat is enough to injure them, but for some people the application of cold works better.

Although not used by everyone, some physicians recommend a spray-and-stretch technique. A vapocoolant, such as ethyl chloride, is sprayed over the tender area to anesthetize it, and then the physical therapist gently stretches the muscles.

Ultrasound or gentle massage following the hot packs is another form of treatment. The hot packs are a method of using superficial heat, while ultra-sound penetrates into the muscles.

The second phase of physical therapy involves exercise. Several studies have shown that an aerobic exercise program is best for those with FM. Aerobic exercises are those that improve cardiovascular fitness; in other words, they improve the flow of oxygen in the blood throughout the body. People with fibromyalgia are often hesitant to exercise, since experience has taught them that pain will follow.

In a physical therapy setting, a mild stretching program follows the applica-tion of heat. When that has been tolerated well, a very gradual active exercise program is begun. It is not uncommon to begin with the simple range of mo-tion exercises recommended by the Arthritis Foundation.

You can then move on to such aerobic exercises as walking, swimming, or bike riding. Not all of the researchers consulted agreed upon how such a pro-gram should be conducted. Some agree with Dr. Paul Reilly and Dr. Geoffrey Littlejohn who believe that although this may make the symptoms worse at first, you should push into the 'pain zone' because you will do yourself no harm by doing so. However, they do suggest that you start gently and persis-tently increase the intensity of the exercise.

The last is the key to remember: "Start gently and increase persistently." If you have been accustomed to an active lifestyle, it is sometimes hard to realize that the most you can start your exercise program with is five repetitions of arm movement or two minutes on a bicycle. That is so little that health-conscious people may question the benefits of doing anything if you must start so low.

But once you have managed to ride the indoor bicycle for two minutes at a time, perhaps twice a day for several days, you will find that you can gradually increase your time. In my initial hospital stay in 1987, I had worked up to three repetitions of some stretching exercises and four minutes on the bicycle. One day I decided that I would increase my repetitions and increase the time on the bike to ten minutes. That night I was in a lot of pain. As a result, I had to return almost to the beginning stages of my therapy. Be reasonable in your expecta-tions for progress.

Several forms of aerobic exercises, including walking and bicycling, can be started at a low level and gradually increased. Exercise is important for a number of reasons. If followed regularly, it brings the body back into a state of conditioning and stimulates the body's production of endorphins. Moderate exercise has also been proven to improve stage-four sleep.

Once released from the hospital or from a physical therapy clinic's outpatient program, it is up to you to continue to practice what you have been shown. It isn't easy to apply hot packs to yourself, but a warm tub bath or regular sessions in a whirlpool or hot tub can easily take their place. You might try using a moist heating pad on low for about 30 minutes. However, intense heat may drain your energy. If you use a hot tub, it is recommended that you don't stay in the water for more than 5 to 10 minutes if the temperature exceeds 104 degrees.

Once you are no longer supervised, it is all too easy to let the exercise slide, even if it's just a day or two. You may feel like there's so much else to do. You're not alone in this behavior. There are indoor bicycles, exercisers, and treadmills gathering dust across the country. But you must push yourself to stick to your exercise schedule because it will take you longer than it does other people to reachieve past improvements. And, of course, there's the chance that you won't be able to reproduce previous improvements.

Jacqueline King has been a physical therapist for 35 years, including eight years in her own private practice. She has seen many people with FM and has watched them struggle to find beneficial treatment. "No one wants to take it on, she says. Too many doctors don't want to spend the time that is necessary, but even beyond that, the health care field is affected by the economics of long-term care. I know this is an extreme case, but I would consider it on the same level as treating cancer. No one is going to die from FM, but they must realize that it is forever. There is no physical therapy or other form of treatment that will cure it or bring total relief.

"There must be a total change in thinking, in lifestyle, and most people are afraid and resistant to change. There must be a commitment to that long-term treatment, not only by the individual but also by the doctor and the health care field, including insurance companies. But there is no guarantee that treatment will bring about relief, and that lack of guarantee leads many doctors to not want to get involved as well as individuals to say 'It's no use. It won't do any good, so why even try to exercise'?"

Having helped a number of people with FM, Ms. King believes individuals must approach their situation from the right perspective. She contends that those with FM face enough negativity from the medical community without contributing to it themselves—even though it is easy to become self-defeatist under the circumstances. Ms. King says, "So much is left to the individual. There's not a lot we can do about the health field, although I believe some changes are going to be made to provide care for those who don't have insur-

Sample Range-of-Motion Exercises

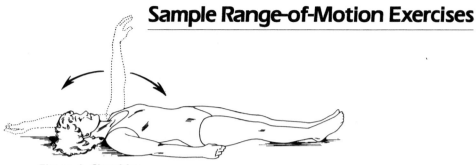

Figure 1. Shoulder

Lie on your back. Raise one arm over your head, keeping your elbow straight. Keep your arms close to your ear. Return your arm slowly to your side. Repeat with your other arm.

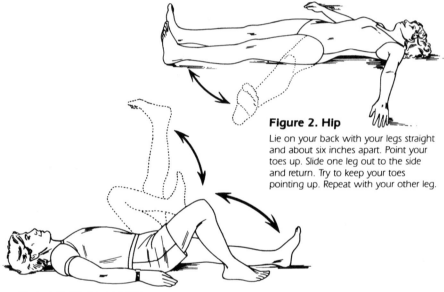

Figure 2. Hip

Lie on your back with your legs straight and about six inches apart. Point your toes up. Slide one leg out to the side and return. Try to keep your toes pointing up. Repeat with your other leg.

Figure 3. Knee and Hip

Lie on your back with one knee bent and the other as straight as possible. Bend the knee of the straight leg and bring it toward the chest. Push the leg into the air and then lower it to the floor. Repeat, using the other leg.

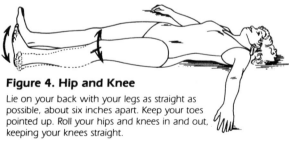

Figure 4. Hip and Knee

Lie on your back with your legs as straight as possible, about six inches apart. Keep your toes pointed up. Roll your hips and knees in and out, keeping your knees straight.

To further strengthen knees, while lying with both legs out straight, attempt to push one knee down against the floor. Tighten the muscle on the front of the thigh. Hold this tightening for a slow count of five. Relax. Repeat with the other knee.

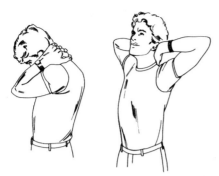

Figure 5. Shoulder

a) Place your hands behind your head.
b) Move your elbows back as far as you can. As you move your elbows back, move your head back. Return to starting position and repeat.

Figure 6. Thumb

Open your hand with your fingers straight. Reach your thumb across your palm until it touches the base of the little finger. Stretch your thumb out and repeat.

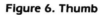

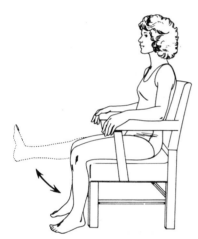

Figure 7. Knee

Sit in a chair high enough so that you can swing your leg. Keep your thigh on the chair and straighten out your knee. Hold a few seconds. Then bend your knee back as far as possible. Repeat with the other knee.

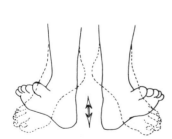

Figure 8. Ankle

While sitting: a) lift your toes as high as possible. Then, return your toes to the floor and b) lift the heels up as high as possible. Repeat.

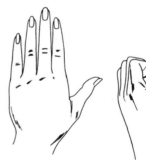

Figure 9. Fingers

Open your hand, with fingers straight. Bend all the finger joints except the knuckles. Touch the top of the palm. Open and repeat.

ance. But people must first decide that they are going to do whatever they can to change their lifestyle and to include exercise. I have to admit that most won't do so on their own. That's why I think they should look for an exercise group, perhaps led by a physical therapist or by someone who can teach them the best way to begin and continue with aerobic exercising.

"It must become a way of life. It takes at least six weeks to see even very small physiological changes. It won't happen overnight and it must be continued."

Decisions about exercise are difficult to make, especially for those with more debilitating cases of FM. My support group includes men and women whose conditions vary from mild to severe. There are several who make it a point to walk a mile or more a day, regardless of their pain. For those who cannot walk a block without severe pain, it is hard to hear these people speak of "walking through the pain." And yet it seems that the authors of the medical journal articles and those who do manage to exercise or carry on their lifestyles with little change fault those who do not enjoy such freedom of movement.

It's almost as if they are saying, "If you would just make the effort, you, too, could do what you once were able to." That is a fallacy that is hard to fight, since it is often expressed in a sceptical tone of voice or with the lifting of an eyebrow. And that belief can add to your guilt and low self-esteem, which in turn can depress you even more.

So what do you do? Struggle to exercise or keep your activity level at an unrealistically high stage, allowing yourself to sink into a continuous cycle of pain, depression, and anger?

You must find the right level for yourself. Regardless of what you have done or felt in the past, at this point only look forward. You know how much FM affects your body, mind, and spirit, which in turn affects your lifestyle and those around you. Working with your doctor and physical therapist or with a group, determine what changes you must make. Start your exercise plan. How much can you do? At what level should you begin? What is best for your condition?

Follow your doctor's guidance. If you begin an exercise program supervised by your doctor and physical therapist, don't stop or decrease your program when released from the physical therapist's care. No one can afford to continue to visit the therapist forever. After you stop going, you must continue your exercises. Try to find an exercise group that is compatible with your program, or organize one with others who have FM. Those who have company in their exercise are more likely to continue the program and accomplish their goals. You also might look into the aquatic programs offered by the YMCA or YWCA.

If you can't find anyone, try it on your own. It's hard, but it can be done. If you are determined enough to make a difference in the quality of your life, you will do it. One important note to remember, you are in this for the long run, so act accordingly.

Osteopathic Manipulation

Recently Dr. Rubin conducted a research study that included the impact of osteopathic manipulation on fibromyalgia and drugs. There were four groups: placebo and no manipulation; placebo and manipulation; alprazolam, ibuprofen, and no manipulation; alprazolam and ibuprofen with manipulation. The results confirmed that the drugs were effective but that manipulation improved people's overall sense of well-being.

Osteopathic manipulation deals directly with the musculoskeletal system, working on the muscles, skeleton, and associated connective tissue. Manipulation aids the body by promoting healing and by maintaining high levels of health, which includes increasing the blood flow, nerve conduction, and lymph flow to and from affected areas. This is accomplished by massaging and manipulating areas on the body to remove any muscular or bone impingement that may be affecting the blood flow, nerve conduction, or lymph flow.

The Effect of
Diet on Fibromyalgia

Many people may wonder if their diet affects their fibromyalgia. Up to this point, research has not found diet to influence FM, although some people experience sensitivity if not an allergy to food. Does that mean then that you can simply ignore food and your diet completely? No, you should strive to eat a normal healthful diet.

One problem that you may encounter is an increase in weight. Some of that may be due to your medicines and some due to decreased activity. Although it has not been confirmed by specific studies on fibromyalgia, it is believed that people with chronic illnesses often have lower metabolism rates.

It is also not unusual for people to eat more as a way of dealing with stress, including the stress of a chronic illness. Not only is extra weight unhealthy, but it puts more stress on the muscles. So many factors can play a part in increased weight, which could lower your self-image even more.

It isn't easy to find yourself in this catch-22 situation, and it isn't easy to make some changes, especially if you live alone and have less energy to cook healthful meals. The Arthritis Foundation recommends the following general guidelines for anyone with arthritis (they also apply for those with fibromyalgia):

- Eat a variety of foods
- Maintain your ideal weight
- Avoid too much fat and cholesterol
- Avoid too much sugar
- Eat foods with enough starch and fiber
- Avoid too much sodium
- Drink alcohol in moderation (Watch this—alcohol often interacts with medicine, producing a dangerous combination.)

The Arthritis Foundation also warns more specifically about combining alcohol and other substances. They explain that stomach problems are more likely to occur if you drink alcohol and take nonsteroid anti-inflammatory drugs or aspirin. Consuming large amounts of alcohol with an acetaminophen can damage the liver. And those are just the dangers of the nonprescription drugs.

Unproven Alternative Remedies

Anyone who has a chronic condition that is difficult to treat can become susceptible to unorthodox or unproven remedies. We've all seen the ads that promise pain relief or an instant cure. Although those directed specifically at people with fibromyalgia are limited, sometimes the promise of relief from pain will tempt the strongest of us.

If there were a cure or a more effective treatment, it would be available to everyone and would be shared by doctors who care for their patients. Always question remedies that promise more than they can likely deliver. Fibromyalgia, like many other diseases and conditions in the rheumatic field, has periods of remission and decreased pain. Such a period can occur independent of any treatment or applied remedy. Just because relief occurs after the treatment does not prove that the treatment brought about the change.

There is no reason to go into detail about unproven remedies, but a word of caution should be in order. Think carefully before you try one. Check with your doctor if someone urges you to try a remedy; do not throw away money for something that may not only be ineffective but also potentially harmful.

The Arthritis Foundation publishes an extremely helpful pamphlet, titled

Unproven Remedies (#4240). The pamphlet is available at no cost and is an excellent resource for anyone considering alternative methods of treatment.

Summing It All Up: How You Can Help Yourself Cope With Fibromyalgia

Dr. Robert Bennett proposed these ten guidelines in *The Journal of Musculoskeletal Medicine.*

Understand the problem

Although we do not know exactly what causes fibrositis, we do know that it is probably the most common cause of musculoskeletal pain. The hallmark of fibrositis is the presence of "tender points"; when pressed, these can cause severe pain.

Increase your overall level of fitness

Most people with fibrositis allow their muscles to become chronically unfit through disuse. Gentle exercise can usually ease the symptoms of fibrositis; however, there is a fine line dividing the amount of exercise that is helpful and the amount that causes an acceleration of symptoms. Each person must determine this dividing line by trial and error.

Slowly resume recreational activities

Although overexertion can cause an exacerbation of symptoms, it does not do any damage to your body. Do not be afraid, therefore, to slowly resume recreational activities. Although you may feel a bit sore the next day, the psychological benefits of being active will probably outweigh the increased pain.

Use heat, massage, or stretching for symptomatic relief of temporary setbacks

These measures can alleviate the symptoms of fibrositis and allow you to continue your activities.

Improve the quality of your sleep

Many people with fibrositis suffer from a lack of deep, restorative sleep. What matters is not how long you sleep, but how deeply you sleep. If, after eight or more hours of sleep, you awake feeling fatigued and very stiff, mention this to your physician. He or she may want to prescribe medication to improve the quality of your sleep. You can also improve the quality of your sleep by going to bed at approximately the same time each night in a room that is not too warm (ideally, the room temperature should be about 60°F [15.5°C]). Reduce extraneous stimuli (such as light and noise) as much as possible and avoid nicotine before bedtime. You can improve your sleep by exercising each day and by not drinking anything that contains caffeine or alcohol, within eight hours of going to bed.

Strive to reduce those stress factors that seem to exacerbate symptoms

Although we are not certain of the exact relationship between emotional stress and fibrositis, it does seem that emotional stress makes the symptoms of fibrositis worse.

Minimize the use of painkilling medications

Medications should play only a minor role in the treatment of fibrositis. Painkilling (analgesic) drugs may be used occasionally to reduce the severity of musculoskeletal pain, but they should not be considered a major method of treatment for your condition. You may become tolerant of any painkilling medication (even aspirin) used for a long period. Consequently, you will need stronger and stronger medications until you risk becoming dependent on narcotic analgesics.

Do not use fibrositis as a scapegoat

Fibrositis never causes destruction of muscles or joints; it is not, therefore, a crippling disease. You should not use fibrositis as an excuse to evade irksome or unpleasant responsibilities.

Do not "doctor shop" for a magic cure
Avoid legal battles over fibrositis

There is, as yet, no evidence to prove conclusively that any type of accident or job-related activity can cause or worsen the symptoms of fibrositis. It is clear, however, that the stress of drawn-out legal proceedings can make your fibrositis worse. Avoid getting involved in such proceedings.

How an Occupational Therapist Can Help

I first met Jean Judy when I was looking for some help in coping with my FM. Ms. Judy, a registered occupational therapist and an assistant professor of occupational therapy at Texas Woman's University in Denton, Texas, helped me in many ways. Her students helped me make the sign that reads "I'd rather be riding a horse" for the back of my wheelchair. And it was she who introduced me to a craft that was not painful to do and that became a new way for me to make money. Do not overlook the possibility of occupational therapy when considering available resources for help.

An occupational therapist's goal is to assist people in continuing to fill the roles they have chosen in life. To accomplish that, a two-objective plan is developed for each role. For a person with fibromyalgia, the objectives are to conserve energy and to develop any adaptations necessary for continuing the chosen role. Due to the inconsistent nature of fibromyalgia, these plans are very individualized.

For people with mild fatigue and pain, for example, the occupational therapist's ideal goal might be to help them to continue working at a full-time job and maintaining their household responsibilities as well. The occupational therapist looks for ways to perform daily activities that require the least amount of energy and place the least amount of strain on the muscles over a 24-hour period, while also encouraging full range of motion in all major joints. Normally, the occupational therapist would conduct a thorough investigation of both the home and the work site. Based upon your individual needs, the occupational therapist suggests techniques and adaptations to the environment that would enable you to conserve energy, making it possible for you to fulfill your roles.

In an interview, Ms. Judy explained the role of an occupational therapist:

> The occupational therapist strives for a balance of work, play, and rest. We believe that a person must have all three. Often, we are able to take an activity the individual was involved in previously and find a substitute that still gives that person satisfaction.

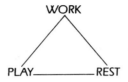

Generally, occupational therapy clinics are associated with hospitals or re-habilitation centers, although there are also some that work with the elderly through home health agencies. Occupational therapy training centers often provide services for members of the community. Check with the colleges and training centers in your area, because they often offer services at discounted rates. The cost of occupational therapy services at these centers varies and is sometimes covered by insurance.

Because occupational therapy clinics are not available everywhere and doctors don't always think about referring people with fibromyalgia to them, it may be hard to find one on your own. The information that follows is just a small part of what you can do to make life with FM easier. If you have access to such a clinic, make a point to check it out. You will be amazed by the amount of practical information that an occupational therapist can provide.

Many times in the past when a certain chore had become very tiring, I considered trying to find a way to simplify it. But because I've always felt that I wasn't really handicapped, I had no excuse to consider making adaptive changes in my daily routine. Few people with FM think of themselves as handi-capped and so view an occupational therapist's help as something they aren't entitled to. This approach is completely counterproductive. You don't have to think of yourself as handicapped. But accept that you do have limited energy and pain that often prevents you from doing what you want and from continu-ing to function. So if occupational therapy can show you how to do necessary tasks while conserving enough energy so that you can still participate in plea-surable, if not essential, activities, then you must tap that resource.

YOU ARE ENTITLED

You don't have to be "handicapped" to take advan-tage of resources that will make tasks easier for you and that will give you energy to enjoy the more pleasant activities in life.

Planning

So where do you start? Begin with planning. If you take the time to plan out your day, your work at the office, and your housework, you will save yourself energy and pain in the long run. Take the time to sit down and write out the various roles that you play in your life. Are you a wife, father, banker, or teacher? Get a yellow legal pad and put one role at the top of each page.

Then on each page list the activities that you do for each role. Let's just start with being a parent. As a parent, you not only handle meal preparation and clothing needs, but you also coordinate your children's activities. Depending on the number and ages of your children, you can often get them to help in ways that will give you more energy. Youngsters can learn to pick up their toys and put them away, saving you from having to bend over thirty times a day to put various toys into the toy box. And think about how heavy toddlers become. How many times a day do you unconsciously bend over to pick up a small child?

If your children are older, they can help out around the house in any number of ways. Sit down together and discuss ways they can help you to conserve energy so you can keep the family functioning as normally as possible.

Priorities

It is important to set some priorities. Sometimes that means giving up or just not doing some things you've always done. It may mean not pulling out the stove and refrigerator to scrub the floor except when you buy a new appliance or move. It may mean that instead of mopping and waxing the floor every week, you give it a lick and a promise during the week and once a month, you give it a top job.

So as you are making out your list of activities, be sure to distinguish between tasks that must get done and tasks that you would like to get done. You will find that there are some jobs that you can skip over in order to conserve energy for more important activities.

Play

Even though people with FM need to have a balance of work, play, and rest, they often decide to ignore the importance of play time. It happens most often when all of your energy is being devoted to making a living. What happens to priorities then? You have to earn a living. But you are only hurting yourself in the long run if you don't include some play in your life. Some people may experience periods of remission, some will have days with less pain, but fibromyalgia is here to stay—don't burn yourself out today.

What kind of play will fit into your altered lifestyle? Occupational therapists try to come up with something that is linked to your activities before FM. For example, if you can no longer ride horses, can you still keep them around? Is there someone who can care for them? If not, have you considered photographing horses? These sorts of options are available for everyone. With your cooperation, your occupational therapist should be able to help you find outlets for pursuing your interests.

Pacing

In order to manage the fatigue that accompanies FM, part of your planning should involve pacing. It is generally easier to talk about pacing than to actually do it. When your mind is intensely focused on a project, you may not want to stop working on it unless you have to. Or it may be that you have always gotten up early and jumped into the less pleasant chores so you could finish them and move on to more enjoyable activities.

For some it may be better to jump in and get it over with, while others will learn that pacing is a necessity. Pacing can be as simple as doing one household chore at a time, such as cleaning the cat box, and then taking a break.

Look at the overall picture. You may have to spread your work over several days in order to accomplish it at all. There will always be some chores that must be done at a particular time, but there may be others that can be shifted.

It is important to listen to your body. The goal, of course, is to do as much as you can and to live a life as full as possible. Sometimes that means working on in spite of the pain and fatigue. At other times, it is necessary to recognize when you need to slow down. Your body will generally give you plenty of warning when you need to slow down or take a break.

You may need to go to bed much earlier than you are accustomed to. This will often have an impact on your social life, but careful planning will allow you to maintain some sort of social interaction. Learn to recognize when you can push yourself and when you should rest.

Pacing should apply to the larger picture of your life as well. If you need to conserve your energy to generate income, that may mean that you don't do a lot of housework or cooking. Consider spending one day preparing meals to put in the freezer. Then you will only have to pop them in the microwave, allowing the time spent cooking daily meals to be used for other purposes. If you still have the energy to cook, it doesn't take much more effort to prepare extra food for use at a later time.

Whatever your situation, pacing can help you maintain a more stable and pleasurable life. Don't dismiss the potential benefits of pacing—you'll be surprised how much it helps to restore peace to your life.

THE 4 Ps

Planning
Priorities
Play
Pacing

General Tips

LIVING WITH
CHILDREN

There are many general tips that help make day-to-day living easier. Your doctors and therapists can suggest additional ideas to supplement these.

If you have young children, try to eliminate bending and stooping as much as possible. This is especially important because most research indicates that FM most often affects the lower back and hips. Try using plastic milk crates as carry-alls. Even if your children are too young to understand the concept of putting their toys away, you can often make the activity into a game, having them put the toys into the crate, which can then be carried to their room or the toy box.

Even with cooperative children, your work may be eased by using such adaptations as an extender. An extender has a long handle that helps you to reach and pick up not only items on the floor but also those above you. It may be just what you need to save a lot of bending and stooping.

A parent may pick up a baby or a toddler over and over again. Although it is often quickest to bend over and pick up the child, stop to think about what stress you are putting on your back. If possible find a chair or stool and sit down first, then pick up the child. If that isn't possible, use your knees and thighs instead of your back to squat down. You may need to steady yourself by holding on to a piece of furniture as you come back up but that's much better than putting all of the load on your back. This holds true for picking up any heavy or awkward item.

Occupational therapists have some extremely helpful ideas about how you can simplify your work, whether it is in the home or outside the home. Let's look at some of the areas in the house where changes can be made. Again, these are just some of the things that can be done. These examples should teach you to look at your environment as if you were seeing it for the first time or from a stranger's viewpoint. Increased awareness will help you find ways of saving energy.

In the Kitchen

Since everyone has to eat, let's begin in the kitchen. If you have teenagers in your family, you might set up a cooking schedule that operates on a rotating basis. Even younger teens can put together a pizza. This arrangement will benefit you and your family; it will generate more family time and prompt your children to learn valuable cooking skills. Cleanup time can be shortened if you have an automatic dishwasher, although some people with FM don't mind washing dishes because the warm water makes their hands feel better.

Of course, everyone is aware of the wide variety of take-out food that is available today. It can become very expensive, even if you are single or live with only one other person; however, it is an option worth considering. The quality and nutritional value of take-out food is steadily improving. Allow yourself the luxury of turning to take-out food when you might have dismissed the option before.

If you like to cook or must cook for a family, there are still some things you can do to make it easier for yourself. Get an office chair with wheels for your kitchen. Whenever you are having trouble standing or getting up and down, use your chair to scoot around the kitchen. Try doing most of your preparation at the table. But if you like to use the counter as your workstation, get a bar stool with a good back on it. Sitting down while doing many tasks is a proven energy saver. Use lightweight dishes and pans. Heavy objects will add to the strain on your wrists and hands; you may even drop them. The same thing goes for pitchers. Heavy ceramic or ironstone pitchers may be attractive and match your dishes, but they're extremely hard to pick up and hold.

Store the items you use most often in convenient places at levels that don't require you to do a lot of extra stooping or stretching. Try to reduce the weight of drawers by removing the items you rarely use and storing them elsewhere. A lot of this may seem obvious, but many people arrange their kitchens the way their mothers did or the same way they've always done it. Now stop and rethink the way your kitchen is organized. What arrangements can you make that will save you steps and energy?

Handling Laundry

Laundry is another taxing chore that plagues everyone, but it can be especially difficult for those with a limited range of motion. However, there are a number of ways you can make laundry less difficult.

If you have to make a number of trips out to the laundry room, consider having two laundry baskets that stay in your bathroom or bedroom—one for clean clothes and the other for dirty ones. Whenever the dirty one is full, you can carry it to the laundry room. Folding laundry, particularly sheets and towels, requires holding up one's arms while performing repetitive motions that cause the muscles in the arms and shoulders to burn and ache. Consider leaving clean sheets, towels, and other laundry that doesn't *have* to be folded in the other basket so you can pull them out whenever you need them.

Making the bed can also be difficult. Make up one side of the bed at a time and, if possible, make sure the bed is clear on both sides so you don't have to do any more stretching and reaching than absolutely necessary. If you choose to fold your sheets, put them in sets, wrapping one in the other and tucking the pillow cases inside. This way you'll have to reach into the closet only one time for each bed. Plastic closet organizers, which have no drawers to pull open, are great for keeping commonly used clothes handy and neat. The items you use the most often should be the easiest to get to.

Ironing demands a lot of energy from the arms and legs. You might want to avoid 100% cotton garments and stick to cotton blends. They combine the benefits of easy care and comfortable feel. If you can afford it, of course, take your clothes to the dry cleaner and allot the saved energy to a more enjoyable activity.

If you have a large family, you might try having several baskets, designated for whites, colors, towels, and other batches of laundry. Place them in the laundry room, if you have room, so you won't have to carry them back and forth. Make each member of the family responsible for placing his or her dirty clothes in the right basket. This will free you from sorting and transporting clothes.

The same idea can be used for items that need to be regularly picked up and returned to their proper place. Set an attractive basket or plastic milk crate in each room. When you finish with something, whether it's a book or some papers, drop it into the crate, and once a week or as often as necessary, make one trip to return the items to their particular place. If you don't already have a system that provides a designated place for everything, this may not be the best time to establish one. Sometime when you are feeling especially good, ask a friend or family member to help you reorganize. Not only do more hands make the work easier, but it's a great opportunity to visit.

Managing Bathroom Chores

With a little creativity you can do several things to ease the burden of bathroom chores. Like most people with muscle pain, you may find that you have a hard time reaching around the bathtub to clean it. Try cutting down a mop handle until it is a length that allows you to easily reach all around the tub. Next, cut a large sponge in half, and then cut a hole in the middle of one of the halves. Fit the half with the hole on the end of the mop handle, making a versatile scrubbing tool that won't force you to get down on your hands and knees to clean the tub. It is also a good idea to quickly run the washcloth over the fixtures and around the flat areas as you leave the bathtub. This is a great habit to develop because it takes only a few seconds once you get down into the tub and saves you from having to return later. Do the same thing at the sink after washing your face or brushing your teeth.

If you have cats and have trouble keeping the litter pans clean, you might consider this: Cut a large plastic trash bag into two pieces and lay the first piece on the floor. Set the clean box on top of that, placing the second piece of plastic in the bottom of the box. You will need a cat box that has a lid to fit over the sides and hold the plastic liner in. (It's a lot cheaper to use a plastic trash bag than to buy special liners.)

Because the sacks of litter are generally heavy, don't lift them and pour littler into the pan. Instead, open the top of the bag and use a large plastic margarine bowl to scoop out the fresh litter. You should also have a "pooper scooper." Try to set the box close to the toilet. Whenever you're in the bathroom, scoop out the solid waste, dump it into the toilet, and flush it away. This way you will have to change the entire box only once a week. Keep the plastic bags, the broom, and scooper in the bathroom to save steps. There are also some long-handled pooper scoopers that would decrease the amount of bending and stooping you'd have to do to clean the litter box.

Juggling Shopping, Errands, And Transportation

You may have always enjoyed shopping and doing errands but now find that such activity leaves you almost sick with fatigue. Getting in and out of the car and walking around the stores can become more than you can manage. The same becomes true for going to art galleries, museums, and special events. It's bad enough to have to give up something you enjoy, but it is more difficult to accept that you are unable to take care of essential business.

You may find yourself reaching a point that you postpone going to the grocery store or running any other errand because it just takes too much energy. If you live alone, it may be necessary to rely on friends to do your grocery shopping and to use the mail as much as possible for other business. You also might consider asking your doctor for a letter that will allow you to obtain a handicap license plate or sticker. The letter will state that your mobility is impaired and your condition is permanent. You may get some unpleasant comments from people who don't see anything obviously wrong with you. Don't take it personally; there are far too many people who do not have a health problem who park in those spots. Being able to park close to the door may make the difference that enables you to get around the grocery store or post office without generating debilitating pain.

What can you do if you still can't get around? It would be easy to give up and stay home, but you would become completely isolated from the world. Consider some of the alternatives. Ask to use the wheelchairs or three-wheeled electric scooters that a number of stores provide. Some department and discount stores have wheelchairs with large baskets, and at least one major discount store has an electric scooter available for its customers. Check with your local merchants.

You might consider renting a wheelchair for special events, if you have someone to push it. However, you should consult your doctor before using a wheelchair for more than special events. You may have no other option than using a wheelchair, but you should never make that decision on your own. Those who use a wheelchair regularly know that it is very important to stretch their hip and leg joints each day. Not doing so is dangerous because it allows the muscles to shorten, further limiting the range of motion. The object of using a wheelchair is to remain active and not to become totally disabled, which is possible if you decide to use the wheelchair permanently.

Another option is using a motorized three-wheel scooter. It still requires some energy to use, but you will be able to do much more than you could without it. Some of the cheaper models run under $2,000 and can be taken apart and carried in the trunk of your car. But before making the investment, be sure you can take one apart yourself and lift each piece unless you have someone else who can do it for you. There are also lifts that can help you get the scooter in and out of your car, but at $1,200 or more, the cost of a lift is also significant. Not all scooters will fit in all cars, so shop carefully.

The Texas Department of Human Services runs a special program, called the In Home Family Support Program, that offers some services for those who are trying to keep working. The program pays up to $3,600 for changes to the home or for special equipment to accommodate a disabled person's needs and provides $3,600 a year for medical care services that are not covered by any other funds. Contact your local Department of Human Services to find out whether your state offers a similar program. Be aware that any program may have a waiting list and require some time before it can respond to applicant's requests.

Even without investing in a three-wheeler, there are several ways you can keep up with your errands and shopping. Some grocery stores offer a delivery service for a nominal fee. Check with the stores in your area to determine which ones provide a delivery service and what their eligibility requirements are. In most communities there are individuals who will run errands, either for pay or on a volunteer basis, for those who can't get out. Look for their ads in your community's newspapers or contact your local United Way or Chamber of Commerce.

There are other simple ways of conserving energy. Let your fingers do the walking! Do all comparison shopping over the telephone, especially when pricing prescriptions. Try to pay all of your bills by mail. Save heavy shopping, whether it's groceries or other goods, until you have help.

When shopping, you will generally find that store employees are very helpful in getting items off the top shelves or dividing up purchases so that no one bag is too heavy. Try not to feel self-conscious or hesitant about asking for help; it will save you from extra discomfort in the end. Today most stores offer a choice between paper and plastic bags. Although the plastic bags are environmentally the better choice (if recycled), they often put a greater strain on your hands and forearms than the paper bags do.

Continuing to drive helps those with FM maintain some independence, but driving and riding often increases the stiffness. In fact, many people with FM become very uncomfortable when they travel for any distance. Any extended travel is usually so painful for them that they have to limit it as much as possible. This can keep them from seeing family members as often as in the past, or from taking part in special occasions.

When you must travel, make frequent stops and allow yourself enough time to walk out the stiffness. If you make sure you are as rested as possible when you start out, you may not have to completely give up travel by car. If you don't have access to a large car with a good suspension system and comfortable seats for such trips, consider renting one. You will find that you will get less tired and will enjoy your stay more if you take these steps to make your travel the least aggravating it has to be.

Transportation And Travel

Public transportation can be extremely difficult for someone with FM. Although taxis can take you door to door, they are generally expensive. Buses and trains are more difficult to use. Many public transportation systems have special features to make them accessible to disabled people, but you may still have to walk some distance to and from them. Some organizations provide rides for those with handicaps. Check your local United Way or Chamber of Commerce for more information.

Traveling by air can be an exhausting ordeal, but there are some techniques you can use to help ease the trip. If you are traveling alone, make arrangements to use handicapped parking and inquire about using a wheelchair. Your airline will have a wheelchair waiting to meet you and take you to your gate. Generally, you will be allowed to board first, although you will probably disembark last. Despite the risk of losing checked luggage, you should carry on as little of your luggage as possible. Remember, you are going to be even more tired at the end of your trip; consider having someone drop you off and pick you up or taking a door-to-door shuttle.

The important thing regarding any travel is to make all of the arrangements ahead of time, taking advantage of handicapped parking and any other special services the airline provides. If you drive to the airport and want to bring your three-wheel scooter, some airlines will check the scooter on through, transfer you to one of their wheelchairs, and then deliver the scooter to you when you reach your destination. The most important thing to remember is to plan ahead. Make your arrangements as early as you can so you can take advantage of any help that will save you energy.

Self-care

There are a number of things that you can do to make taking care of yourself somewhat easier. If you find that you can't hold your arms up long enough to continue your daily grooming routine, you need to think about adopting a "look" that requires less effort. Men may opt to grow a beard, eliminating the strain caused by shaving. Women might consider another hairstyle—one that doesn't require the use of a curling iron or rollers. Try a casual style that is easy to care for, yet flattering. Your self-confidence is already damaged—pick a look that you like and feel good about. Don't just assume you'll have to sacrifice your attractiveness for ease.

There can be several other difficulties involved in taking care of yourself. Because of the muscular pain, you may have a hard time getting up and down to use a toilet. When you're out in public places, always take advantage of the handicap stalls. Taking a bath often requires some advance planning to determine the best and easiest way of getting in and out of the tub. Without becoming overly anxious about using the tub, try to be more aware of the dangers of falling. Put no-skid strips on the bottom of the tub. Install a bar on the wall or side of the tub that you can hold on to when getting in and out of the tub. Get a short stool to sit on while in the tub, so that you won't have as much trouble getting out.

If you have a shower, you might consider using a shower stool and secure support bars. If you put the bars in yourself, make sure they are connected to the supporting boards and will hold your weight if you slip and start to fall.

Remember that bathing with all of its accompanying activities such as rinsing the tub first, running the water, washing, shaving, and dressing can be exhausting. Again, plan ahead to conserve energy.

If there are activities that you can no longer manage to do, such as shaving the back of your legs or washing your hair when your neck and shoulders hurt so bad that the very thought of bending over makes you shudder, there are some steps you can take to help. Try adding a handle to your razor. It can be something as simple as part of a curtain rod fastened to your razor handle with strapping tape. You need to measure first to get it the length you need, and you may need to keep a second razor handy for areas that you can still reach easily.

When washing your hair, try pushing a chair up to the sink so you can kneel and take some of the strain off your muscles. It won't relieve all of the strain, but even having your hair washed at a salon may lead to some uncomfortable moments.

Consider bathing every other night instead of every day, unless you've been particularly active, and have as much as possible prepared ahead of time. Take everything you will need into the bathroom at some point earlier in the day.

A bar stool with a back on it will allow you to sit at the bathroom mirror to put on your makeup or to shave. If you have a dress that zips up the back and has one point that you just can't reach, get a piece of twine, tie a knot in one end, and run the other end through the hole in the zipper. Holding the twine, pull the zipper up, slip the twine out of the hole until you are ready to take off the dress.

Try to wear slip-on shoes instead of those that have to be tied. If you have to wear ties regularly, try loosening the knots, instead of completely untying them, just so that you can pull your ties on and off. This way you can just pull one over your head and tighten the knot, avoiding the added muscle strain involved in completely tying it.

Rest

As you already know, rest plays a vital part in the effort to conserve energy. But there are several important aspects of resting. Some sort of break should become a part of your regular schedule. At home, you might try a variety of different methods. At least one session of relaxation therapy or meditation would be a good start (see Chapter 8). Or you might just lean back in your recliner, if it seems to take some of the pressure off of your lower back, and stay there for 10 to 15 minutes.

At other times, you might need to stretch out on the couch and actually fall asleep. Generally, when this happens, your body needs the extra rest, so don't try to fight the sleepiness. You may need to take the phone off the hook or plug in the answering machine so you won't be disturbed. Taking regular short breaks may reduce the need for long deep naps.

Many people never really think about furniture and its comfort until they develop chronic pain. Sometimes it takes trial and error to find things that can make you more comfortable. You should make sure you have a good supportive mattress and a pillow that will support your neck rather than your head. If you are having trouble with your arms and shoulders, support them with extra pillows. When you lie on your side, the natural weight of the arm not supported by the mattress can pull it down, making you more uncomfortable. Resting it on a spare pillow significantly eases this discomfort. Your doctor or physical therapist may be able to recommend a good pillow that properly supports your neck. You may also want to purchase an egg carton pad for your bed.

When sitting, try to elevate your feet. Try putting a footrest under the kitchen table, your office desk, and even your computer table. It can be almost anything from a cinder block to an upholstered stool but should be about $5\frac{1}{2}$ or 6 inches high. If possible, sit in a recliner or use a footstool so you can get your feet up. And when you sit on the toilet, prop your feet on the bathroom scales.

It is extremely important that you have furniture that provides you with good support and lets you sit comfortably. A good bed promotes restorative sleep, and a good chair eases muscle strain by encouraging proper posture. By using comfortable furniture and frequently changing position, it is possible to avoid stiffness.

Adjusting
to the Changes

Fibromyalgia takes you into a new world. Whether you have been there for years as you searched for a diagnosis and effective treatment or have just arrived as a newcomer whose symptoms appeared only recently, this world is probably one filled with anger, fear, frustration, and pain.

If you are like many people who have been misdiagnosed and struggled through treatment after treatment that brought no relief for your pain and fatigue, you're probably feeling more than a little anger. You have a right to be angry. In today's advanced technology, we have come to believe that doctors know so much that almost anything should be easily diagnosed and treated. There should be a pill for whatever ails you. But all the shoulds in the world won't change the fact that medical researchers still have a long way to go before they can recognize and treat every medical condition that arises.

Actually, fibromyalgia is only one of hundreds, if not thousands, of medical conditions that doctors have a hard time diagnosing and treating. But does that fact make your life with FM any less painful or easier to live with? No. And you shouldn't expect it to. No matter how many times you are told to be thankful that it is not life threatening or crippling, it doesn't make facing each day of pain and fatigue any easier. Your life has changed. You are the one dealing with the pain and fatigue. You are the one who must live with that 24 hours a day, everyday.

So what can you do? Withdraw into your secluded world of FM? It may be tempting. But you don't have a choice about having fibromyalgia. You can only make a choice about how you are going to live with it now that it is part of your life. One step in beginning to cope might include adopting "The Serenity Prayer."

When I resigned from my last full-time job, I wrote "Serenity, Courage, and Wisdom" on a small blackboard and hung it where I could see it every day. As you will learn, each day is a new day, and even though you may believe you

---

THE SERENITY PRAYER

God grant me the serenity to accept the things I cannot change, the courage to change the things I can,
and the wisdom to know the difference.

---

have conquered the anger, fear, and depression, the battle is never really won. Some days are easier and some days are harder, but every one must be faced— faced and lived.

It would be so easy to resign from life, to sit down in a chair and refuse to do things that you know will cause pain. It may be easy, but it's not something that you *can* do. You cannot give up. There is something within all of us that does not even want to acknowledge giving up. Regardless of the pain and fatigue, you need to spend the rest of your life living life to the fullest, whatever that is for you. Whether it's the bookkeeping system or the parking arrangements, people tend to resist change.

And now you are faced with changes that you don't want to make, changes that are being forced on you. For instance, as an adult you may have never taken a daytime nap, even though you walked around in a fog of fatigue, because you were determined to keep going. Now you may find that a short nap, or at least a brief rest on the couch, will enable you to put in more work time in the long run. Look at these changes as a positive way of making life easier for yourself.

Coping With the Anger

When I realized that I would no longer be able to get and keep a full-time job, it made me angry. It also scared me. After all, I'm single and must support myself. It had been hard to manage financially when I was working full time. What was going to happen now that I couldn't keep that full-time job? The thought frightened me, causing the fear and anger to feed on each other in a never-ending cycle. For over four months, I walked around wanting to put my fist through a wall.

There are productive ways of expressing anger. And, as most people know, it is much healthier to express the anger than to keep it buried. You must learn and incorporate the safe ways of expressing the anger so it doesn't smolder and eventually erupt. Besides the physical cost of holding in the anger and the stress of controlling an outburst, you may also damage a lot of relationships.

Coping. *Webster's New World Dictionary* defines *cope* as "to fight or contend with *successfully*." Presumably, you are learning as much as you can about fibromyalgia, which is an indication that you have chosen to cope. Coping with any chronic illness is a constant fight. It takes a conscious effort. Living with fibromyalgia is not easy. Your course of action must be deliberate and planned. And even though there is always the element of uncertainty, you must develop alternative strategies that you can use to meet that uncertainty.

The first step, again, is making the decision that you are going to live as well as you can. The second step is forming a partnership with your health team and establishing goals. And the last step is facing the emotional impact of the changes you are experiencing.

Handling the Changes in Your Life

Whether you have already confronted the changes in your life or they are just now appearing, you need to recognize several facts. Everyone fears and resists change. It isn't unusual to be nervous when you start a new job. But even when you are excited and looking forward to it, there is still an element of reluctance to make the change. How often have you heard someone say, "But that's the way it's always been done" when asked to make a change?

By expressing your anger, you have recognized your legitimate right to get angry and decided that you aren't going to let that anger become a disruptive force in your life. But remember that although you have the right to feel angry, you don't have the right to make yourself and everyone else around you miserable. On the other hand don't burden yourself with guilt about being angry in addition to the anger. Whether you express it by having a good crying spell or by throwing something, you must be able to let it go. Your fibromyalgia won't go away, nor will most of the circumstances change, but your ability to live with them will improve.

Will one expression of anger, one crying spell or the satisfaction of seeing something break, end all of your anger? No. You will still get angry, particularly when there is something you want to do but don't have the energy to do or cannot do because the pain is too bad.

Don't misunderstand, it isn't easy to learn how to vent your anger in an acceptable, healthy manner. Your first reaction may be to find a physical release for your anger. But when this sort of activity can severely aggravate your condition, this is not a realistic option. Don't be afraid to go to a psychologist or counselor who can help you find effective and appropriate ways to release and cope with your anger. You may need some help.

Feeling All Alone

Anyone with chronic pain may have many sleepless nights. You may have them regularly at certain times, or you may not have any trouble at all. Sometimes, you will be so tired that you can't imagine why you can't sleep.

How do you manage to get through those long hours? Try reading. Reading will help you get through the night, and it can also help you cope with the pain, by diverting your mind.

Loneliness may plague you more often these days. You may feel removed from everyone else. No one understands just how tired you are or just how much the pain hurts. You feel isolated and alone. But there are others who do understand. They may have fibromyalgia or some other chronic illness. Realizing that you are not alone is one of the most important things you can do. You may find others within a support group or even in your day-to-day contacts who are struggling with the same experience. However you find them, these friendships will help to ease the loneliness.

Dating and Personal Relationships

Dating is another important issue for single people with fibromyalgia. When you are single and the sole breadwinner, you have to fill several roles. For a single person, the role of breadwinner is the most important because you must support yourself, regardless of your condition. But that is not all, you must also be a friend, as friendships are essential to your mental stability. And you are a family member, whether or not you have children, if you still have parents or brothers and sisters. Time spent with your family can still be socially fulfilling, but you also need the joy that comes from social interaction with others.

Make the effort to get out of the house periodically even if it's only to meet a friend for lunch or a glass of tea. The change of scenery will renew your spirit, and the outing doesn't have to be expensive.

Where is there time and energy for a social life that includes dating? Although it may seem as if there is no time for that, it is important that you at least make the effort. You may not feel up to a night on the town either. If you have always loved to dance, it can be disappointing to have to sit out every song. And late nights may be totally out of the question now. How do you continue to meet new people? What do you do about dating?

Try to get out at least once a week or every two weeks. If you don't have the energy for dancing, go to hear a special performer. Of course, you will want to be well rested before you go, and try to make sure you have a comfortable chair to sit on. You may not be able to sit through an entire show, but it is a wonderful way to enjoy the music without feeling left out of the activity.

What do you say about your fibromyalgia to a potential romantic interest you've just met? Although you may want to get your health condition out in the open immediately, you don't want to pour it all out on a first meeting or even a first date. Unless he or she has asked you to go hiking, there's no need to bring it up until you both decide that you want to see more of each other. You will need to find the line between using a lot of "I can'ts" and refusing to discuss the reasons behind your limits.

If your relationship grows, some of your limitations will naturally become apparent. If the person you're dating is very involved in physical activities, it is best to be realistic and honest about your condition from the beginning of the relationship. If continuing intense physical activity means more to your partner than continuing a relationship, let go of the relationship before you become involved in a painful situation. For anyone who is more interested in getting to know you better, your fibromyalgia won't matter—it will just be a part of you.

Sometimes you may feel as if you just don't have the time and energy to even consider dating. That is all right, too. After all, you must set your priorities. But don't use FM as an excuse to hide from a relationship, and don't use it to manipulate someone into a relationship. Sometimes people feel that FM has stripped them of their attractiveness and choose not to be open to meeting someone new. Concentrate on the aspects of your attitude and appearance that you can do something about. Don't agonize over those you can't change. You have to make the effort to meet new people, regardless of the complications involved. No one will come knocking on your door to improve your social life. Remember, you need a balance of work, play, and rest.

Sex and Intimacy

"My husband has stopped approaching me about sex. I'm just too tired after a day's work and then coming home to cook supper and clean up."

"It hurts for someone to even bump into me, much less some of the affectionate hugs and touching my wife and I used to enjoy."

Many times couples find it very frustrating to handle a chronic pain condition and still maintain intimacy in their relationship. Even today, many health care providers are hesitant to address the topic unless their patient brings it up. And yet anyone who considers asking a doctor about sex and intimacy may rightfully worry that such questions will be dismissed.

No one can question the importance of sex and intimacy in marriage, yet what can you do when sometimes even a light touch brings pain? How do couples who have always had a very physically intimate relationship cope with the reality that such touching may cause one partner pain? It wouldn't take too many sessions of painful contact before a couple becomes too afraid to touch.

And if just touching causes pain, what about lovemaking? Does a couple have to give up their sexual relationship completely? If the marriage wasn't overly strained before, this could overburden it completely.

Even if your doctor is reluctant to discuss it, there are sources of help and information. Your occupational therapist can provide plenty of information on the physical aspect of relationships. An occupational therapist doesn't become involved with the dynamics of a relationship but can give guidance in choosing times and possible positions that would put less strain on affected muscles. Or your doctor may be very willing to talk it over with you and is only waiting for you to ask.

If you are uncomfortable speaking with someone directly, there are a number of books that can be helpful. Check out the health and self-help section at your bookstore or the local library. The Arthritis Foundation publishes a booklet on sex and arthritis titled *Living and Loving,* which also offers some helpful hints. See the appendix for other titles that give tips for coping with this aspect of chronic health problems.

Although spontaneous intimacy is usually preferred, carefully planned moments of intimacy can be just as exciting if approached with the right frame of mind. After all, if you have taken the time to be well rested, the experience is more likely to be enjoyable than if you have to cut it short because you ran out of energy.

Depending on the location of your pain, different positions can prevent lovemaking from adding to the stress or strain on those muscles involved. Such positions can be found in some of the books published (see the Appendix), but you shouldn't feel limited by them. Together you and your partner can explore the possibilities. A warm bath to ease your muscles and a dose of analgesics taken in time to provide some relief might help to make intimate moments as painless as possible.

Although many couples make love in the evening, those with FM enjoy no benefits for doing so. By evening, their fatigue has caught up with them, especially if they have been active. Mornings may not be the best time either because you may awaken stiff and in pain. For many, the best time to make love is late morning or early afternoon. Experiment and don't be afraid to be innovative because it won't damage your body or accelerate your condition. After all, you want to nurture your marriage as much as you can under the circumstances.

If you are single and not involved in a long-term relationship, it will be more difficult. A great deal will depend on the person you date and his or her attitude toward your fibromyalgia. At a time when sexual issues are discussed more openly, you should be able to talk about this with your partner. Some choose not to become involved in a relationship so they won't have to worry about confronting these issues. Be careful about taking this approach. A supportive partner can bring so much joy to your life that you will be glad you didn't avoid an intimate relationship.

The important thing to remember is that intimacy is a vital part of love, and sex is a part of intimacy. Of course, it's possible to be intimate without physically expressing your love, but if you and your partner are patient and plan a bit, sex can still be a part of your relationship.

Facing the Fear

Fear is very much a part of learning to live with a chronic condition. It may not be unusual to experience fear that is so strong it causes extreme panic. In the beginning, it may be difficult to believe that there is a limit to such fear and panic. You may fear the consequences of being unable to support yourself or of being incapable of meeting your commitments as a member of a family. The fear may also be rooted in knowing that constant pain is going to be a part of your life from now on.

Just as it is acceptable to feel anger, it is acceptable to feel fear. But you cannot let it completely command your life. Again, you must exert some control, control that you may feel that you will never have again. Much of the fear expressed by those with FM is related to the loss of direction of their lives. There are some things you will never totally control again, and that is why it is so important that you make the effort to maintain whatever activities you can. Fear, particularly fear of change, is understandable and acceptable. But do not let it and the other emotions you are experiencing rule your life because they will only contribute to your symptoms.

FM's Effect on Your Self-Image

All of us carry around an image of ourselves inside of us. That image is not how others see us, but how we see ourselves; it shapes all our actions and thoughts. All of the things that make up the person that is you are encompassed in that self-view. Your physical shape and size, the color of your hair, your eyes, your skin, and the way you dress and carry yourself are all factors. The roles that you play help to determine that self-view in both positive and negative ways. If you have a successful career and a happy marriage and home life, you will generally see yourself in a positive light.

Deep within you, you have certain expectations of yourself—certain ideas that determine how you behave. If for some reason, you are unable to meet the expectations that not only you have, but that others have for you, your self-view will be affected. Fibromyalgia can seriously affect that image. Perhaps you can no longer provide for your family financially and making love with your wife may have become too painful. Or perhaps it has become impossible for you to plan special outings for your family because you're never sure how you're going to feel. Or maybe you can no longer keep working at a job outside your home, which is necessary for your family's financial welfare. Being unable to fill these roles will inevitably have a detrimental effect on your self-image and happiness.

Fibromyalgia affects more women than men, and most of those women are in their 30s or older; the average age of women affected is mid- to late 40s. So, many women with FM came of age before the women's liberation movement began and were taught that they would be judged on the quality of their housekeeping. It may not have been an overt lesson, but it was still one that they absorbed.

Yet many women, if not most of us, also work outside the home. Almost any woman's magazine contains articles that demonstrate that regardless of the post-1970s raise in consciousness women are still the ones doing the housework. Most of us come home from a 40-hour-a-week job to another full-time job of laundry, child care, errand-running, and housework.

This routine is enough to burn out a woman who has a normal energy level, so what can it do to someone who runs on half a tank, *if* she's lucky? Many of us still associate the image of self with maintaining a house. And when we can't measure up to our own standards, even if our husbands or partners don't insist on such standards, our self-esteem is affected.

When you add the problems associated with keeping an outside job to the low self-image as a housekeeper, parent, and spouse, it becomes a grave situation. When you add that to the pain and frustration of a poorly understood, difficult medical condition, you are left with the potential for some serious psychological problems.

Because many of you have been told that your pain and fatigue is due to psychological problems, you most likely don't want to hear that there may be such problems. In this case, they are caused by your pain, other symptoms, and the changes that are taking place in your world. And that is only natural. But how are you going to deal with them? You must realize that you are grieving and that you must work your way through the grief process, emerging with a more acceptable view of yourself.

The Grieving Process

Grieving occurs whenever we lose something or someone. We realize that it is natural to grieve over death and many also realize it is part of the divorce process. But is it all right to grieve because you have fibromyalgia? Haven't you lost something? Your health? This is usually more apparent to someone who has only recently developed the symptoms of FM.

It may have been only a few months ago that you took that great hiking vacation or that you could spend all day shopping at the mall, ending the day with a special dinner for two. Now you find it difficult to stay at the grocery store long enough to get your usual supplies and just the thought of physical exertion leaves you out of breath.

Whether you were that active or not, by the time you accept fibromyalgia, you have lost a lot. It may be the ability to work as long as necessary to put your ideas into action. It may be horseback riding and owning your own horse or taking long hiking vacations. It may be climbing the corporate ladder to reach the position you always wanted. Whatever you have lost, recognize that legitimate loss has occurred in your life.

These losses are tied into the grief process. It is natural for you to experience grief. And it is all right to grieve. But you must not let yourself get stuck in any of the first four phases of grief. Denial or isolation, anger, bargaining, depression, and acceptance are all the stages of grief, and you must go through each of them. Often people also experience guilt for feeling these emotions.

It is a very personal journey, and no two people experience it the same way. Some will remain stranded in the first stage of shock, while others may move rapidly through the first two stages of denial and anger only to try bargaining or fall into the abyss of depression.

Human nature cushions us somewhat from the first blow of grief by staging a period of denial during which we may try to isolate ourselves from the truth. This gives us time to begin the healing process of grief. The length of time you spend in any of the stages isn't as important as the fact that you make your way through the process and come to terms with your loss. It is natural to initially deny your FM, to believe that it really won't have an impact on you. That isn't much of a problem to someone who needs only a mild analgesic to control their pain, but it is unrealistic for those who must alter their lifestyles.

Use common sense in facing your loss. And be gentle with yourself. After all, you didn't deliberately get fibromyalgia. You can be angry at the FM, but you don't have any reason to be angry at yourself.

Usually, in any loss there is a period of shock, almost to the point of numbness, which is the body's way of easing you through the first period. The second step is denial, accompanied by a sense of loneliness. For many who have FM, that sense of aloneness is eased when we realize that there are nearly ten million Americans who have fibromyalgia to some degree. They've got lots of company.

Anger generally follows. The worst aspect about being angry about FM is that there is no definite object to be angry with. If someone makes you mad, you can direct your anger at them. But in FM, there is no clear-cut culprit. No one knows yet why FM strikes, and although some can point to a particular incident that seemed to set it off, it just crept up on many others. There is no one and nothing to blame.

You might get angry at the doctors, but it's not their fault either. You may be angry because someone failed to diagnose it sooner or refuses to take you on as a patient, but doctors are only human too. Getting angry at them will only affect your relationship—a relationship that has a tremendous impact on your well-being.

The next step is usually a period of bargaining. You will begin to believe that if only you act in some specified way, then everything will be okay. You try to bargain your FM away. Most people realize fairly quickly that this approach is not going to work.

Depression usually follows bargaining. However, some people move through these phases in different order and even experience some of them more than once. Depression can become very serious and often creeps up on you. You have a right to feel sad, and it is while coping with depression that you come face to face with the reality of your chronic condition. You are most vulnerable during the depression stage.

Sometimes the depression is minor, particularly if your FM is mild or in remission. At other times it can suck all of the light and happiness from your life. Depression is the one stage in which you need to maintain a constant support system. Quite often it occurs for only a short time, yet there are other times when it blocks out any potential for a happy future.

STAGES OF GRIEVING

Denial/isolation
Anger
Bargaining
Depression
Acceptance

It is important for you to recognize the symptoms of depression, to realize that they are a natural part of the grieving process and of living with a chronic health problem. Realize now that you can build a support group that will help you when it seems as though tomorrow and a better day will never come.

When we grieve for a lost loved one, we eventually reach a stage of acceptance. We know that that person is gone forever and that we must go on. In your grieving process, you will also arrive at a state of acceptance, although it will not be quite as permanent as it is when losing a loved one.

SIGNS OF DEPRESSION

- Feelings of sadness that last far too long
- Major changes in sleep habits, resulting in more or less sleep
- Listlessness
- Poor concentration
- Major changes in eating habits
- Sense of worthlessness
- Severe feelings of guilt
- Lack of interest in sex
- Thought of or attempts at suicide

Quite often, your grief will be cyclical. There are times when you will feel you have come to terms with the reality of life with FM and won't expect to feel anger, guilt, or depression again. But then a time may come when you want desperately to do something and realize you can't, because the price you will pay in pain, fatigue, and, most important, in time lost at work, is too high. And so you will return to the cycle of anger and depression.

But you do learn to overcome the emotions that go with grief. No one can stay wrapped up in them forever. Once you have made your first trip through those emotions, you know that you can handle whatever comes—you know that you'll live through them and emerge from the experience as a stronger person.

Coping:
Where to Go for Help

Once you start looking around, you will find that there are many resources, both professional and nonprofessional that you can tap to help make your life more comfortable and easy. Depending on the level of intensity of your fibromyalgia, you may or may not need all of the following resources. But even those people with minor problems will find resources that can be of help to them.

How Psychiatrists and Psychologists Can Help

Many people with FM want nothing to do with these health care givers, but you should try to keep an open mind about them because there are many ways that they can help. Both psychiatrists and psychologists deal with psychological problems, yet only psychiatrists are physicians and are qualified to prescribe and regulate the antidepressants that are used to treat FM and depression. Unfortunately, depression can, and usually does, become part of living with a chronic pain condition. And it is nothing to be ashamed of, although too many people refuse to acknowledge it and seek help. Obtaining a psychiatrist's help is important under these circumstances.

Many psychologists specialize in helping people to live with chronic pain. These specialists are trained in the alternative methods of coping with pain and do much more than just one-on-one counseling. Many of them facilitate group therapy sessions, and teach self-hypnosis, relaxation therapy, and biofeedback.

Because traditional medicine provides little relief from chronic pain, many people feel the need to explore nontraditional methods of achieving relief. Within the last 20 years, some of these methods have gained wide acceptance. There are a number of alternative methods of treatment that directly involve the person seeking help. The methods are generally taught to the client, who then continues the practices or procedures independently. Usually, though not always, it is a psychologist who does the teaching. I learned my early relaxation therapy from a nurse practitioner who had a Ph.D. in counseling and pain control, but it was a psychologist who taught me the principles of biofeedback.

The concept of conscious mental control used for stress management in the form of relaxation therapy, self-hypnosis, and biofeedback can be traced to ancient times (even though the modern world is credited with developing the technology that makes biofeedback possible). These techniques all focus on the tie between the mind and the body and allow the individual to exercise a measure of control.

ALTERNATIVE METHODS OF COPING

Relaxation Therapy
Self-Hypnosis
Imagery
Biofeedback
Stress Management

Again, just as with drugs, physical therapy, and manipulation, some alternative treatments work for one person, while they do not relieve another person's pain and fatigue. It is also true that these methods work in cycles. They may deliver results for a while, but then the effectiveness wears off. Often if you try them again later, you will once more experience a period of positive results. Some techniques may have an initial high cost, while others may involve no more than the price of a book and the time investment. You must decide if you are willing and able to make whatever investment is required.

Behavior modification is often used in the treatment of chronic pain because there is so little else that is effective. Pain is the body's natural warning indicator, informing the mind of tissue damage or illness. Acute pain follows an injury, operation, or illness that causes damage to the body, but it is short term. Once the underlying cause is removed or healed, the pain disappears.

This is not the case with chronic pain. Fibromyalgia has become one of the best examples of chronic pain syndrome. No underlying cause can be found, yet the pain is severe and lasts for months or years. Although a great deal of research has been conducted on pain, its perception, and its methods of treatment, it is still a mystery.

One of the theories on fibromyalgia is based on the hypothesis that something has triggered the central nervous system and shifted its sensitivity into "high gear," causing those with FM to have a very low pain threshold and tolerance. In other words, it takes less of a stimulus for you to feel pain, and you generally have more difficulty handling it for any length of time.

It is helpful to accept and understand that there is an actual link between the mind and the body. It is commonly accepted that stress can be a prelude to high blood pressure, a heart attack, or an ulcer. It is also necessary to accept its role in FM. The alternative treatments are based on the recognition of the effects of stress, regardless of whether those effects surface in organic changes.

Stress commonly causes people to "tense up," contracting their muscles into hard knots. This comes from the body's instinctive "fight or flight" reaction to danger. In a healthy body, the accompanying flow of adrenalin leads to muscle contractions. Since muscle spasms are already a troublesome factor in fibromyalgia, this only compounds the problem.

Many times we react to the pain in our bodies by tensing up even more, unconsciously adding to the problem. In order to obtain some relief from this cycle of muscle pain, you need to learn to relax the muscles involved. Learning to do this requires a conscious effort, because most people are not familiar with the individual muscle groups. One method of relaxation teaches people to clench each group of muscles and then relax them so that they are aware of the difference. An example would be clenching the jaw and holding it that way for two to four seconds before releasing the tension. The difference between muscle contraction and relaxation then becomes quite obvious. Unfortunately, for many people with fibromyalgia, this process only makes the pain worse, so it may not be the best relaxation method for everyone.

If you choose to attempt relaxation techniques on your own, Dr. Herbert Benson at Harvard Medical School explains how to do so in his book, *The Relaxation Response*. However, Dr. Benson recommends that anyone using the book for specific health purposes should do so under a doctor's supervision.

The basic concept of relaxation therapy is simple. It is based on bringing the body to a state of complete relaxation by emptying the mind of all worries and pressures. The general method for achieving this is by going into a room by yourself with no distractions (such as a stereo or television). Make yourself as comfortable as possible in a chair or recliner; some people lie on a bed or a couch. But when you use the technique during the day, you don't want to fall asleep; you should just work toward becoming gently relaxed.

Close your eyes and let all of your thoughts just float out of your head. It is not always easy the first few times you try it, but you don't want to aggressively push your thoughts away. If thoughts keep intruding, just imagine yourself gently releasing them so that they drift out of your mind.

The first time you attempt relaxation, you may not be able to tell exactly which muscles are clenched or contracted. This is a good time to find them by consciously tightening and then loosening them. Begin with the muscles at the top of your head, then in your forehead, and on to your eyes. Feel the muscles in your jaws, let them relax so that your mouth feels almost ready to drop open.

Progress to your neck and shoulders and down your arms to your hands and fingers; move all the way down your back. Then come back to your chest and stomach. Move down to your thighs and then down your legs to your toes. There is no rush, no need to hurry. Take your time, so that you feel each group of muscles relax.

At this point you will experience a sense of warmth and lightness throughout your body that almost feels like you are floating. If you choose, you can use imagery, enabling you to travel in your mind to some restful place. It can be anywhere that you would enjoy being—a warm beach, an open meadow, or even a soft, pillowy cloud. Stay there until you feel a sense of peace and rest emanating throughout your mind and body. Then slowly and gently return. Again, don't let outside thoughts intrude on your return; let them just drift away.

The entire experience should take about 10 to 15 minutes, and when you are finished, that sense of peace should follow you back into your regular day. It won't relieve all of your problems or pain, but it will ease some of the muscle spasms that increase your pain.

From the very simple exercise above, such methods as self-hypnosis and biofeedback have developed. Many people don't believe that they can be hypnotized, and even though some can't be, most find they make good subjects. If possible, have your doctor refer you to someone who can teach you the basics and determine the best method of hypnosis for you.

Costs vary depending on the area and the availability of hypnotists offering their services. Sometimes, university psychology departments offer clinics with reduced rates or provide services through a rehabilitation program. Check with the colleges or universities in your area. As with other alternative methods of treatment, sometimes the methods only work for a while before becoming ineffective for some unknown reason. For example, some people who use tapes their psychologist made for them for self-hypnosis often switch to different sets of tapes when they feel that the old set is losing its effectiveness. This approach also applies to medical treatments. So instead of feeling that you have tried everything and found nothing that works, try returning to previously used treatments.

With the help of personal computers and special software, biofeedback has become much less expensive and is now a feasible option for many more people. The concepts of biofeedback and relaxation are very similar.

In biofeedback the amount of tension is measured with small electrodes that can be placed on your finger and forehead, or on any set of muscles that you need to learn to relax. The equipment used in the early 1970s required the use of big complex machines, which were attached to electrodes that measured the temperature in the muscles. You learn to lower your temperature and relax your muscles by concentrating. The tension in the forehead registers as a series of beep tones that are very fast when first hooked up but that slow as you learned to ease the muscles. Regardless of the specific setup a particular psychologist uses, the goal is the same: to teach people that they do have some control over their bodies and that they can learn to relax tense muscles.

Stress management could be incorporated into the techniques for relaxation therapy, self-hypnosis, and biofeedback. But it is also much more. Stress management is designed to work for your overall life including your work, health, familial situation, and more.

The theory is to identify what stressors are present in your life and how they affect you. The next step is to develop ways to relieve some of them and to find methods of coping and living with others. Stress is defined as a mental or physical tension or a strain. You already know about the effects of stress on your body, specifically on your muscles. Having fibromyalgia is stressful. The condition is inherently full of uncertainty. One day you may be able to do your job and get a great deal accomplished, yet there is no indication of why another day is so different that you can only do the minimum required to take care of yourself. This type of uncertainty is frustrating for you, and for your family and friends, who see no reason why the days turn out the way they do.

Pain itself is stressful. When it goes on without true relief day after day, you began to lose the ability to cope with it. So many of the feelings that accompany FM only add to your stress.

Sometimes everything in your life seems determined to become difficult at one time. Just when your FM is flaring up and you have less energy and more pain, a major crisis occurs at work. Just when you think you have that under control, the washing machine breaks down and floods the laundry room when your budget is stretched so tight it's screaming. Or the transmission goes out on the car that you were trying to make last another year.

Everyone's life has times like this. No one's life always runs smoothly. So why should we expect it to change for us just because we now have fibromyalgia? We can't. What we can do is to try to be prepared for such times and use a psychologist's help to get through them. It might even be worth the time and money to join a group therapy session for a while. If possible, join one that is composed of others who are experiencing chronic pain. There won't always be one, but you can try.

It is difficult for many people to tell their deepest fears and emotions to someone that they have not had a personal relationship with, even if that person is qualified to help them regain some stability. The idea of sharing one's deepest feelings with a room full of strangers seems even worse to most people. Participating in a group therapy session may seem impossible for you, but particularly if it is a chronic pain group, it may be the best thing you have ever done for yourself.

You will find out that you were not alone in being afraid, angry, and in feeling less confidence in yourself. You will also discover how others cope with their emotions. Usually there is a set number of weekly sessions, such as a six-week period of sessions, and you will save money on the cost of counseling by meeting in a group.

It is by participating in a group like this that you can learn how to build up a support system for yourself. This is particularly important if you have no close family; you need to find others who will listen when you need to talk and who understand what you're going through when you need to cry. This is an informal arrangement and one that should be flexible enough to meet your personal needs.

One of the studies on fibromyalgia found that people with FM seem to experience more stress from the hassles of daily living than they did from larger stressors like death or divorce. If this theory is proven, it will indicate that we need to look for ways to help us cope with everyday hassles, which can include anything from the crime rate to traffic to running errands.

Of course, using your time and energy effectively will allow you to accomplish more, but old habits are hard to break. If you feel better, you may slip back into pushing yourself more than you should. Sometimes, you will succeed without triggering any problems and sometimes you won't. Remember, you are in this race for the long run.

The Role of Self-talk

Self-talk is another area in which psychologists are especially helpful. Self-talk can affect your well-being just as your self-image does. As conscious beings, there is constant communication going on in our minds. That self-talk is closely tied in to our view of ourselves, even though most people aren't really aware of that communication or of its implications.

The voice within you is based on all of the things you were told as a child growing up. If you grew up in a home full of love and caring, you were most likely supported in your endeavors as you became an adult. But if your home was one that was not supportive, if it was what is now called a dysfunctional home, you probably need to evaluate what that voice is telling you.

If you grew up with a very low sense of self-worth, your inner voice may be adding to that because your FM prevents you from fulfilling your roles in life, whether that is of spouse, parent, money-earner, or all of those. If pain prevents you from working, your feelings of uselessness may become confirmed.

It may be necessary to employ a psychologist to help you cope with your negative self-talk, or you may simply need to become aware of what you are saying to yourself. You need to be able to take an honest look at yourself to determine whether you are truly doing the best that you can under the circumstances. If you are doing your best, then you need to accept that. If you find that you're not doing as well as you could, then you might find that a program of positive self-talk will help.

Motivational speakers advise their listeners to repeat a positive sentence or two a number of times during the day. It can't hurt to develop one or two of your own. Good examples might be, ''I know that I am doing the best I can'' or ''I will make two contacts with someone outside my home today.''

Of course, you must be honest with yourself. You must *really* be trying to do the best you can. Self-honesty is sometimes difficult and painful. But it is always necessary. You must believe that you are wholeheartedly trying to live and work in spite of the pain. Only you can really know whether you are surrendering to the pain or living your life in spite of it.

—— ■ ——

When Fibromyalgia Affects Your Work

Most people today work outside the home because they must satisfy financial needs and because such work provides them with a sense of satisfaction, a sense of worth. This is also true for anyone with fibromyalgia, but for many of those people, working is not so easy. When you wake up exhausted, there isn't a lot of energy for charging into the working world, even if the desire is there.

Regardless of the type of work, you must have enough energy to handle both the negative and positive aspects of it. Whether you are an assembly-line worker, a secretary, or an executive, you must manage demands on both your physical and your emotional health. There is no indication that fibromyalgia worsens with time, but sometimes there are aspects of the working world that make it seem as if it does. Sometimes fibromyalgia has very little impact on a person's ability to work, but sometimes it forces a person out of a current job or out of work completely. Few studies have been conducted to determine how many people with FM have disabilities that affect their work, but the studies that have been done show that the number runs between 5% and 20%.

In an ideal world, everyone would have adequate health care and doctors would at least be able to maintain the status quo, but many Americans do not have health insurance or the money to pay for regular health care. That means that often, a person's condition does worsen for lack of that care. Although the health care crisis is drawing more and more attention, it is unrealistic to expect any quick solutions.

Whatever your situation, it is important to realize the importance of working, not only for the financial aspect but also for the feeling of self-worth that it provides. If you are still employed, do as much as possible to retain that work. There are three basic ways to handle your work situation: retain your present job, change jobs or careers, or find an alternate means of income if you must quit full-time work.

Again, try to continue to work, whether it is in your present job or a new one. If your FM is so bad that you can no longer work at someone else's schedule, there are many ways you can still earn income—don't give up.

Retaining Your Job

Even if you enjoy your present job and your fibromyalgia allows you to keep your position, your employer may have misgivings about your capabilities. Although they may be extreme cases, some people have been forced out of their jobs. This is a reality that you must prepare for and possibly confront. Quite often, employers do not want to retain employees who have a high absentee rate or who are unable to produce at top speed.

Everyone would like to believe that employers recognize the value of retaining employees who have been with the business for sometime and know their jobs well. And everyone would like to believe that the company would be willing to make some effort to keep those employees by adjusting the working environment or the job structure. Such companies and employers do exist. Only you know if you work for one.

Telling your supervisor about your fibromyalgia could mean that you will be eased, or even forced, out of your job. But there is also a chance that you won't. Sometimes if a person has worked for a company for a long time, the company will be willing to work with that person. It would be a good idea to discreetly check on your company's past actions in similar cases if you can. If you have worked for the same company for some time, you may already know about your company's record in situations like yours. Do be cautious about voicing your concerns too quickly. If you leave your job, do so whenever it is best for you. Let it be your decision, not the decision of your supervisor or the company's management.

Looking into the Americans With Disabilities Act

If you are unsure about your legal rights and the way your company is handling your situation, read the Americans with Disabilities Act. Depending upon the severity of your fibromyalgia, the Americans with Disabilities Act, (ADA) may help you retain or obtain employment. The act addresses the issues of employment and public accommodations for those with disabilities. Employers with

25 or more employees will be covered starting July 26, 1992, and those with 15 or more will be covered beginning July 26, 1994. A booklet titled *The Americans with Disabilities Acts, Questions and Answers,* published by the Civil Rights Division of the U.S. Department of Justice, explains the ADA's purpose in the following terms:

> *The ADA prohibits discrimination in all employment practices, including job application procedures, hiring, firing, advancement, compensation, training, and other terms, conditions, and privileges of employment. It applies to recruitment, advertising, tenure, layoff, leave, fringe benefits, and all other employment-related activities.*

> *Employment discrimination is prohibited against "qualified individuals with disabilities." Persons discriminated against because they have a known association or relationship with a disabled individual also are protected. The ADA defines an "individual with a disability" as a person who has a physical or mental impairment that substantially limits one or more major life activities, a record of such an impairment, or is regarded as having such an impairment.*

> *The first part of the definition makes clear that the ADA applies to persons who have substantial, as distinct from minor, impairments, and that these must be impairments that limit major life activities such as seeing, hearing, speaking, walking, breathing, performing manual tasks, learning, caring for oneself, and working.*

> *An individual with epilepsy, paralysis, a substantial hearing or visual impairment, mental retardation, or a learning disability would be covered, but an individual with a minor, nonchronic condition of short duration, such as a sprain, infection, or broken limb, generally would not be covered.*

> *A qualified individual with a disability is a person who meets legitimate skill, experience, education, or other requirements of an employment position that he or she holds or seeks, and who can perform the "essential functions" of the position with or without reasonable accommodation. Requiring the ability to perform "essential" functions assures that an individual will not be considered unqualified simply because of inability to perform marginal or incidental job functions. If the individual is qualified to perform essential job functions except for limitations caused by a disability, the employer must consider whether the individual could perform these functions with a reasonable accommodation.*

Reasonable accommodation is any modification or adjustment to a job or the work environment that will enable a qualified applicant or employee with a disability to perform essential job functions. Reasonable accommodation also includes adjustments to assure that a qualified individual with a disability has the same rights and privileges in employment as nondisabled employees.

Making Your Job a Little Easier

Even without the ADA, there are many things you can do to make your present job easier. Again, this is something that is very individualized and depends on your job and your degree of FM, but here are some general ideas you can think about.

If you work in an office and are able to consult with an occupational therapist, ask him or her to visit your job site and evaluate it. Your occupational therapist will review the work environment first, identifying anything that could be easily changed. Do you work under an air-conditioning vent? This is something that could aggravate your FM. Can you or your desk be moved? Can a screen or partition be set up to block the direct flow without making everyone else in the office uncomfortable?

Is your chair comfortable and does it provide adequate support? What about your desk? Is it the proper height? Do you find yourself in a strained position as you work? Do you have a footrest under your desk to ease the strain on your leg and back muscles? Is there a chair you can sit on or a stool you can rest one foot on if you have to make more than a couple of photocopies? Switch feet if you stand with one foot on a stool and one on the floor for even five minutes. This alternately relieves the strain on your legs and back muscles.

Do you have a lot of walking to do? Can you plan your day's activities so you won't have to move around a lot or sit in one position for too long? Unfortunately, every job cannot be planned in advance. Many times activity in the workplace is based on uncontrollable factors such as customer's needs, telephone calls, and those little emergencies that seem to pop up continually.

Is there any way that present equipment can be adapted to ease the strain on muscles? If you spend a lot of time on the telephone, think about getting a phone rest, a speaker phone, or a headset.

Two types of strain—physical and emotional, or stress-related—can occur in the work environment. Although physical strain might be eased by using a more comfortable chair or moving the furniture, emotional, or stress-related strain, is not as easy to avoid. Generally, this type of strain is generated by the demands of the job or by your coworkers. Because stress is one of the factors that can exacerbate the symptoms of FM, you may need to re-evaluate your job and your commitment to it.

If you are constantly challenged by your job, find it exciting, and don't feel exhausted every night, don't leave it. A boring job, even if it is easier, would most likely cause more problems. But if you find that you can't maintain the daily pace, that you are completely drained every night, or that you snarl at the kids each evening, you need to think about changing jobs.

Sometimes it is possible to move to a position that generates less stress without leaving your employer. Depending on your career goals, you may feel left out of the corporate challenge. This may be a case where you have to re-evaluate your priorities.

Quite often, stress at work comes from coworkers. Many times office politics and interpersonal relationships can make you miserable. It seems like there is always someone who continually passes the buck or who likes to keep the office stirred up about something. If you face such a situation, you must determine how much this type of stress affects you and your FM. Keep in mind, however, that this sort of stress will often exist where two or more people work together, so changing jobs will not always eliminate it.

Making the Transition from Full-time to Part-time

Sometimes it becomes necessary to give up full-time work and take a part-time job. Adjusting their hours and the demands of the job will enable many people to continue working and earning money, even if it is on a lesser scale. That might be the best thing for you, particularly if your FM has become seriously debilitating. The change to part-time work allows you to keep your foot in the employment door and set your own pace, so that FM does not have such a major impact on you and your lifestyle.

If you can afford it and have a family, this may be one way to increase the time and energy you have for your family. By easing some of the physical strain of full-time work, you can schedule rest periods and activities with your family.

Often, it is also possible to leave a stressful full-time job for a part-time job that is much less demanding. There are many part-time positions that provide income yet do not have the stress that a full-time job does. Whether you decide to continue to work part-time depends on your needs. If you are not facing serious financial problems, part-time work may give you the best of both worlds by allowing you to earn money without having to cope with the added pain and fatigue your full-time work caused. However, be aware that part-time workers are not usually offered the same benefits that full-time workers are. Make sure you understand the terms before you make any major change in your employment.

Changing Jobs

What if you have tried, but have been unable to keep your job, because the company is unwilling or unable to work with you or because your fibromyalgia is just too severe to let you continue in that job?

One possibility is to take some time off work to take care of yourself and possibly to find a new job. Another option is retraining. This is probably going to be necessary if you have been doing physical labor that you can no longer do. How and where do you find retraining? What does it cost?

Depending on your financial circumstances, you might consider going to a community college or university and making a complete career change. Even though recent budget cuts have affected many of the programs that offer grants and loans to students going to college, there is still a lot of help out there, and it's possible that you may qualify for such help. Most colleges and universities also have a center for handicapped students. These provide assistance needed to meet class requirements and to access all facilities.

You must realize that pursuing a new educational goal often adds to the stress level. If you haven't been to school in some time, the period of adjustment may be especially stressful. For some time now, most colleges and universities have seen an increase in older students attending classes for the first time or returning to the classroom so they can change careers. Most institutions are aware of the difficulties older students encounter and will generally work to ease the transition for those students. But only you can decide if you are able to handle the requirements of attending classes at a university or a community college. If you decide to return to school, be sure to take advantage of the institution's career counseling. Most career counselors are great information sources and will be glad to help you find new employment opportunities.

If your fibromyalgia is serious enough, there is another possibility. Each state has a vocational rehabilitation agency. The goal of these agencies is to help the handicapped secure and maintain jobs. Those eligible for this help have disabilities ranging from orthopedic deformities to mental health problems, alcoholism or drug addiction, internal medical conditions, and more.

Not everyone with FM will be eligible, but if you have had problems working because of your fibromyalgia, you should contact the nearest office to determine your eligibility. The rehabilitation centers' services may include: a medical, psychological, and vocational evaluation to determine the nature and level of your disability, job skills, and capabilities; counseling and guidance to help you and your family plan proper vocational goals; limited medical treatment if it is possible to mend the disability; some assisting devices that will stabilize or improve your function on the job and at home; training in a trade school, business school, college, university, rehabilitation center, or even on the job; and selective job placement services. Check with your state rehabilitation program for its eligibility requirements and services.

Fibromyalgia is a condition that may present some problems for a person seeking help. The lack of documentation, such as lab tests and X rays, is one of the problems. Because of this, it is very important that you have complete reports from your doctor documenting your illness and any job loss that has occurred due to FM. One of the other problems is that FM often has periods of increased pain when work may not be possible. Remember, each case is decided on an individual basis. If you believe that you qualify, or even if you think you do, contact your local office or state rehabilitation program.

Turning to Self-employment

Even if you can't work at a part-time job, there are ways to earn money. For the person who is willing to try new things and to learn, there is always a means of earning some money. However, you must be realistic and understand that it is unlikely you'll be able to make enough to replace your full-time income. Most important, remember that you must be willing and you must maintain a positive attitude so you can recognize opportunities and take advantage of them.

One of the best aspects of self-employment is that it will allow you to set your own schedule so you can pace yourself. Sometimes you will need to push yourself, but then you will be able to take the time afterward to recover. Remember, fibromyalgia does not cause your body to deteriorate; you will not be damaging joints and muscles by being active. You will have limited endurance and will probably pay for your actions with some increased pain. But compare that with not earning any income, and you will discover that even though it hurts, you will have gained more than you've lost.

How do you find work you can do that will earn you some money? First you need to sit down and look at yourself and the skills you already have. Not only do you have to consider your education, work experience, and interests, but you must also evaluate the strength of the economy in your region. Realistically assess the market for your services or goods.

Take a step-by-step approach to this process. You may want to enlist a career counselor to help you do this. First, list your education. What do you already have that can be useful in self-employment? Is there any way you can use your skills to work from your home, at your own pace?

If you have at least a master's degree, you may be able to teach as an adjunct instructor at a local college or university. Pay, of course, varies with the college and the locale. Teaching as an adjunct is not quite self-employment, but usually if you are not teaching more than one class and your students have access to you before or after class, the only time you are officially committed to is the actual class time. All of your preparation and grading work can be done at your own pace.

If you do not have the education required, sometimes work experience is considered adequate. Many junior colleges and private colleges hire people from within the community to provide instruction based on their hands-on experience in a specific field.

If there are no openings with colleges in your area or you don't have enough education, there are a number of other ways that you can still teach. They do not usually pay as well, but they do provide some income. Check into continuing education departments at colleges and public schools, as well as recreation departments of the city. They offer classes in almost anything that they believe people are interested in, from writing and photography to calligraphy, from flying an airplane to gourmet cooking.

If you have sufficient experience, and can establish a reputation, you may be able to conduct classes on your own. Even in small towns there are people who wish to learn new skills or arts. There are classes in writing, music, theater or drama, dog obedience, personal finances, painting, games, dancing, and quilting. If you have a special skill, it's likely that others in your community are willing to pay to learn it. Of course, you must set reasonable prices and a clear agenda for the classes. You may have to rent a hotel meeting room to hold your classes, but you may also be able to use your church or civic organization's facilities for a minimal fee.

Although many people believe that writing books is for someone else, you may have special knowledge or experience that you can share with others. The ratio of nonfiction to fiction books published each year is about 40,000 to 5,000, or eight to one. Many of those nonfiction books share personal experiences; others share knowledge. Take the time to go to a well-stocked bookstore and do research. People are hungry for knowledge. What special knowledge do you have to share?

Even if you do not have the ability to teach others or to write, there are many ways that you can earn money. Many hobbyists have earned a living by expanding their activities and creating goods to sell. Many craft malls will display and sell handmade items for a flat rental fee without requiring you to spend long hours at a booth. If you can tolerate spending a day at a booth or table, many local and regional fairs charge an entry fee and provide space where craftspeople can sell their work. You must obtain a tax number from the state comptroller's office because you will have to pay sales tax on the items you sell. But by doing so you will receive a certificate that enables you to buy your supplies at a reduced rate. Many people earn enough money during the preChristmas period to live on for an entire year.

Some other ways of generating income include these possibilities: establish a secretarial, typing, or bookkeeping business at home; start a video or photography business; produce a newsletter for a church, organization, or club; begin breeding purebred dogs or cats; step up a genealogy service; serve as a consultant or do freelance work, sharing your knowledge directly. Working in direct sales is another way of earning money. For some people, selling cosmetics, soft goods, or jewelry has become an enjoyable, low-stress method of drawing an income.

The most important thing to remember about self-employment is that there will be no time clock to punch and no supervisor peering over your shoulder. To earn money, you must be motivated and a self-starter. It is possible to fit this in as a way of working in spite of your fibromyalgia but you must learn to know when to rest and when to push yourself.

Check with your local Chamber of Commerce for information about SCORE, the Service Corps of Retired Executives. They can offer free assistance to those who are considering going into business for themselves. Another source for help is the Small Business Administration.

What If You Need Help?

Sometimes it turns out that no matter how hard you try, the threat of financial problems becomes overwhelming. Where can you turn for help? As discouraging as your situation may seem, there are some resources that you might turn to.

Check to see if you have a disability insurance policy through your place of employment. Generally, these policies cover only a limited period, but that may be all you need to get back on your feet. Carefully read any such policy; don't immediately dismiss it just because it appears to offer limited coverage.

Apply for Social Security disability benefits. As previously explained, it is difficult for those with fibromyalgia to qualify for benefits. But each case is judged individually, and they do take into account each applicant's level of education and line of work. Even if you don't think you have much of a chance of getting the benefits, apply anyway and take it as far as you can.

What if you are like many people with fibromyalgia who slip through the cracks? You are able to earn some money but not enough to live on, and that amount disqualifies you for many forms of assistance. If you find yourself at this point, you should know that there are still some resources available and people who want to help.

If you're worried about paying your basic bills, there are a couple of sources that can help you locate funds to pay the electric bill before they cut it off or the rent before you are evicted. Although finding those agencies and associations that are willing to help can be a frustrating search, it doesn't have to be.

On the local level, approach the United Way office, the Information and Referral Services, or the Chamber of Commerce office to acquire a list of human service agencies. Check the telephone book for other human service organizations in your area. Now many phone books list such agencies in a special section in the front of the book.

If you belong to a church or temple talk to your pastor or rabbi. While some churches still provide help on an individual basis, many have turned their contributions over to an interdenominational ministries program. Contact the social welfare office at your local hospital; you don't have to be a patient to get referrals from them for sources of assistance.

Sometimes, depending on the region, there are additional programs available to you. You can be directed to them by contacting the regional department of human services office. Each state does have a department of human services with regional offices throughout the state. The personnel at these offices can put you in touch with programs originating with federal, state, county, or city agencies. Each program will have its own set of guidelines and eligibility requirements.

Asking for and accepting help, whether it is transportation to the grocery store or the doctor's office or money to pay this month's rent is often very difficult. But many of these programs were set up to help those who are unable to manage, particularly because of their health. There is nothing that says you will have to use their help forever. But at least during the rough times, try to find out if you qualify for assistance. Later on, when you are back on your feet, the funds can be passed on to someone else in need.

Establishing
Support Systems

"No man is an island" is especially true for anyone who must face a chronic health condition. Those of us with chronic health problems may be more likely to fall into deep depression and believe we can't endure. But we don't have to face life with fibromyalgia alone. Sometimes we may feel that we would be better off alone, but that's not true at all. We need family and friends. And we need to know that others share our experiences.

The ideal support system would include family members, friends, and a support group, supplemented by such organizations as the Arthritis Foundation. All of these groups play important roles in helping you maintain your well-being. Make an effort to establish such a system for yourself.

The Role of Family

Ideally, the family is your first line of support. After all, these are the people who care about you the most. It would be wonderful if family members always responded to our needs in a positive way. But quite often that doesn't happen. Spouses may feel angry and frustrated; children may not understand.

Most of the time, the love and respect that develops during a marriage will carry a couple through the rough times. Unfortunately, the very nature of fibromyalgia puts a strain on even good marriages. Because FM is so unpredictable, many times plans have to be canceled or changed. When a couple starts out, they usually bring certain expectations to the marriage. If one member can no longer carry out those expectations, such as working and bringing in a full-time income, the goals of the marriage must be re-evaluated and often reset. Sometimes, even spouses can begin to doubt the severity of the pain and fatigue. Spouses may also resent having to assume responsibility for activities that their partners previously handled.

An interesting study, conducted a number of years ago, found that in a large percentage of cases, when women contracted rheumatoid arthritis after marriage, their husbands were unable to cope with the situation and left the marriage. This did not occur when the man developed rheumatoid arthritis. If the woman already had rheumatoid arthritis when the couple married, the problem did not arise as often.

Perhaps because it is still so new, no such study has been conducted on those with fibromyalgia. But *any* chronic health condition adds stress to a marriage. If you think your FM is affecting your marriage, seriously consider marital counseling. If the love and respect is strong enough, you and your psychologist will find a way to keep the marriage together. You need that sense of support and love even more now that you face FM.

Sometimes a person with a chronic condition develops a *sick role*. A sick role is the term for using one's condition to manipulate others or to avoid fulfilling responsibilities. Sometimes this behavior is unintentional and is often reinforced by family members and friends who care about the person and want to protect their loved one from additional pain and suffering. The person with FM as well as the family and friends must realize that, while there are limitations, life must still be faced and lived responsibly. How can you avoid falling into a sick role? Increased awareness helps. If you are aware of the potential for it, you are less inclined to develop one.

Conscious or unconscious manipulation only complicates an already complex situation. A certain amount of pain and fatigue inevitably accompanies FM. But if you try to totally retreat from this pain, you will also retreat from the joy of life. You must find fine line between living and ignoring the real limitations of your condition. This is not easy. It requires commitment from both partners as well as some "tough love." Quite often it takes the help of a skilled counselor and a lot of compromise and communication among all those involved.

If a marriage is already on shaky ground, a chronic condition may completely destabilize it. That pressure could be the impetus that ends the marriage, or it could also become the catalyst for rebuilding a marriage full of the love and caring it was founded on. Although no one knows in advance which marriages might fail under the burden, there are some steps you can take to keep a relationship together.

Communication and counseling, as already mentioned, provide a good beginning. Just as education about fibromyalgia is important for the person who is learning to live with FM, it is also important that the spouse and family members learn about it. Once a diagnosis is made and a treatment plan developed, the family needs to become involved. Some activities and responsibilities may need to be shifted, temporarily or permanently. Goals and priorities should be reviewed. It is not necessary to immediately change everything around you, but as time passes and you understand FM's long-term impact better, you can discuss your options as a family.

Your children need to be involved in this process, but be careful not to force them to assume an adult's role while they are still children. Many times when a parent becomes ill, the oldest daughter is expected to assume her mother's responsibilities and the oldest son becomes responsible for his father's duties. If there is any way to avoid this pattern, you must find it. It is one thing to have children perform some role in maintaining the home, and it is another thing to pull them prematurely into adulthood. Talk it over with your family, so all members are familiar with the desirable changes and can work together to prevent damaging patterns from developing.

When establishing your support system, don't overlook the importance of your family's role. Many people find that they never would have been able to come to terms with their FM without the support of their loved ones. Adversity often draws a family closer together, bringing out new facets of each individual's personality that may not have been evident before. Turn to your family for help—you may be surprised by the inspiration and strength they give you.

The Importance of Friends

Thank God for friends. Friends are an important part of everyone's life, but they are especially important if you are single. As with family members, friends must work to maintain their relationships. More important, friends may be more likely than family members to walk away from someone they feel is using them. And yet there are times when a friend will be there for you when a family member is not.

Communication is vital to people. We all want and need to discuss the things—good and bad—that are happening in our lives. If you have a family, it is probably natural to share with them. But if you live alone, you must reach out and communicate with someone. This is when the telephone can become a lifeline.

Even if you are stuck in bed or at home for a while, the telephone is your doorway to the world. It enables you to contact someone whether you need some specific task done or just someone to talk to.

You don't have to tell all of your friends all about your fibromyalgia. Some will want to know all about it, and others will want to know only a little. So try to be selective in how much you say. For some, it may be difficult to accept that you look good even though you feel terrible. When those you aren't particularly close to ask how you feel, chances are pretty good that they don't want to know the specific answer. Just say something like, "I'm feeling better today" or "I didn't have such a good night" and move on to another subject.

With those who really care and really want to know, you still must be careful to avoid boring them to tears or continually dumping your troubles on them. Try to follow a few rules about your friends. Do talk to them about your fibromyalgia, but try not to let it monopolize the conversation—there are many other things to talk about. They need to know that you care about them and want to know what is happening in their lives and careers and how their families are doing. If your friends are married, recognize that their spouses and families are their first priorities and try to always respect that.

If you need to talk to someone, try not to call on the same person too often. Your friends may insist that they don't mind, but you don't want them to feel that you call only to complain. If you need to talk, call one friend today and another one tomorrow or the next day. And always make an effort to call or meet your friends just to talk, as you would do in any healthy friendship.

Try not to impose on them for favors. If you can manage to take care of something on your own, do so. If you can't manage by yourself, try to ask for help only if it is convenient for another person to help you. You want to remain as independent as possible, but don't carry it too far.

Many times your friends are glad to help, they just may not be sure what they can do. You will find that the world won't come to an end if a friend has to do something for you. Actually, it gives them an opportunity to express their love and caring for you. Don't deny them that expression. Try to remember the good graces of friendship. Always *ask* for help, don't command or demand. Say thank you and mean it. And whenever possible, do something for your friends in return. There will usually be something that you can do, even if it is only listening when they talk about their problems.

Sometimes as you try to come to terms with your fibromyalgia and its effect on your life, you may feel that your friendships are one-sided, with you doing all the taking and none of the giving. But you should know that you have some-thing to share as well. Just as you often need someone to listen, your friends and family members occasionally need a listener, too. For many people, talking about their problems is one of the most effective ways of coping with their experiences. That's not always true for others, but sometimes the need to talk to a sensitive listener does arise.

Even with fibromyalgia you should try to maintain as wide a range of interests as possible, and try to have friends who share some of those interests. By having more to talk about than just your health, you invite stimulating and enjoyable conversation.

Remember the old adage, "If you want to have a friend, you must be a friend." Even when it seems your world has narrowed to just yourself and your fibromyalgia, remember that those around you have something that is equally important in their lives.

Another Resource: Support Groups

No matter how much your family and friends love and support you, unless they have fibromyalgia, they really don't know what you are experiencing. They may have been with you through the frustrating months or years while you sought a diagnosis and treatment, but they can't experience the pain, fatigue, and emotional impact of chronic pain.

Joining a support group can connect you with people who have the same special needs that are not met by other support systems. The knowledge that you are not alone makes it much more bearable. When others have already walked the path that lies before you, they may be able to share information that will make your journey easier. This is true whether you are coping with a divorce, a career change, or a health condition like FM.

Some support group members need to talk with others and to vent their frustration. Frustration is a word commonly used, for good reason, among people with fibromyalgia. The problems of getting a correct diagnosis, an effective treatment, and facing the day-to-day challenges of living with FM generate a lot of frustration. For many people, talking eases those feelings, and just knowing others have the same experiences helps. On the other hand, some support group members just want to get the group's newsletter and stay informed.

Many support groups across the country share and distribute a lot of information. They stay abreast of the increasing number of articles that are appearing in medical journals and general periodicals. Several newsletters on fibromyalgia also provide information for support group members. One of the best is a quarterly newsletter from California that provides updates on the newest developments and interviews with researchers. Although education is the first step in developing a health plan, not enough educational material is available for the layperson.

Support groups may create the potential for members to focus on negative aspects rather than on ways of improving their lives. When you meet to talk about your fibromyalgia (or any condition), there is a chance that the meeting will turn into a gripe session instead of a healthy exchange of positive feelings. There may be people who do not attend to have a positive experience. Instead, they attend so they will have the chance to talk about the severity of their case and to monopolize conversation.

Many doctors are hesitant to sponsor support groups because past experiences have proved to be unproductive. They don't want their patients to continually focus on the negative or to dwell on their problems. They are right, because it is unhealthy to do that. It is best, when first organizing a support group, to adopt some guidelines that will prevent each meeting from turning into a "pity party." Sometimes it isn't easy, especially when you have members who feel the need to control sessions, but if everyone is aware of the reasons for the guidelines, you can work together to prevent the negative results from overwhelming the positive ones.

Ron Burks, a psychologist in Wichita Falls, Texas, has this important piece of advice for anyone, whether they are in a support group or among their friends: "Get off the pity pot." It's okay to talk about your problems with someone. Sharing them can divide them in half. But don't stay in that mode of behavior. Put a limit to the amount of time you are going to feel sorry for yourself. For that time, allow yourself to be unhappy, to recognize your sorrow. Then move on to something more positive. After you've done this, life will be a whole lot sweeter and your friends will still want to come around. But most important of all, you will feel better emotionally. And you will want to be around yourself for the 24 hours a day, 365 days a year, that you must live.

SAMPLE GUIDELINES FOR
FIBROMYALGIA SUPPORT GROUP

STATEMENT OF PURPOSE

This group is designed to provide people with fibromyalgia and other interested people the opportunity to talk freely about problems, concerns, and frustrations, and to share information, encouragement, helpful hints, and support. Through your participation in this group, you can learn more about fibromyalgia, or fibrositis as some still call it, and get ideas about what can be done to ease its effect on your life.

WHAT HAPPENS AT THE MEETINGS?

Meetings are open to the public and may include talks, with question-and-answer sessions, given by various medical experts, general discussions among members, and special entertainment. Educational sessions may include films or seminars on problems of daily living. Generally, the meetings last about 1½ hours.

GUIDELINES FOR THE SUPPORT GROUP

1. We are a group of people with a common bond, sharing our concerns, feelings, experiences, strength, and wisdom.
2. Our discussions are designed to foster positive attitudes and are directed toward solutions. We share our problems, but we do not dwell on them.
3. We listen, explore options, and express our feelings. We do not prescribe, diagnose, judge, or give medical advice.
4. We know that what we share is confidential.
5. Our leaders are not "the experts," and most sharing of ideas will come from us.
6. We each have the opportunity for equal talking time or the right to remain silent; we can share as much or as little as we want.
7. We actively listen when someone is talking and avoid interrupting and participating in side conversations.
8. We encourage "I" statements, so that everyone speaks in the first person. We stick to our own experiences and avoid generalities.
9. Our meetings supplement and do not replace medical care.
10. We do not promote quackery or provide specific medical advice.
11. We each share the responsibility for making the group run smoothly.
12. Having benefited from the help of others, we recognize the need to offer our help to others.

Courtesy of The Fibromyalgia Association of Texas, Inc.

Nonprofit Organizations: An Invaluable Resource

Organizations such as the Arthritis Foundation in the United States and the Arthritis Society in Canada, the American Chronic Pain Association, and the

California Network of Self-Help Centers are other sources you can approach for support.

Even though fibromyalgia is still relatively new, the Arthritis Foundation and the Arthritis Society include information on it in their regular publications. In the United States the national publication is the bi-monthly *Arthritis Today*. Area chapters generally publish newsletters that are also available to anyone interested. The Arthritis Foundation prints a small pamphlet on fibromyalgia, and a number of other organizations produce pamphlets that cover subjects of interest to those with FM (see Appendix).

The mission of the Arthritis Foundation is to support research to find the cure for and prevention of arthritis and to improve the quality of life for those affected by arthritis. It carries out this mission in a number of ways. The foundation sponsors the Arthritis Aquatic Program, self-help courses, and arthritis clinics for low-income people; provides a wide variety of literature, a physicians referral list, seminars, a speakers bureau, and support groups; and sometimes has a loan closet for home medical equipment. They also help with the "Kids on the Block—Arthritis Program," which teaches school-age children about arthritis. People with FM can also use these services and programs.

The Arthritis Foundation also sponsors fund-raising activities to help cover their expenses and to go toward research.

What You Need to Know

What is fibromyalgia?

Fibromyalgia is considered a non-articular (affects muscles, ligaments, and tendons, but not joints) rheumatic condition. It is often referred to as fibromyalgia syndrome because at this point, we don't know what causes it so it can not be considered an illness.

What are some of the other names fibromyalgia has been called?

Fibrositis, fibromyositis, tension myalgia, myofibrositis, interstitial myofibrositis, myofascial pain syndrome, myofascitis, musculoskeletal rheumatis, muscular rheumatism, nonarticular rheumatism, tension rheumatism, psychogenic rheumatism, psychophysiologic musculoskeletal reaction, and conversion reaction.

What are the symptoms?

The primary symptom is widespread pain that often feels as if it comes from the joints, but fibromyalgia affects the muscles and the locations where ligaments attach muscles to the bones. Pain, like the aching that accompanies a bad case of the flu, can occur all over the body in addition to the presence of sharp pain in specific spots. Tender points at specific locations around the body are extremely sensitive. Fatigue, stiffness, and non-restorative sleep are also symptoms.

What are the criteria for a diagnosis of fibromyalgia?

In 1990, the American College of Rheumatology established a set of criteria for the diagnosis. It includes a history of widespread pain, lasting over three months, that occurs on both sides of the body and above and below the waist. At least 11 of 18 established tender points should be extremely painful when pressure is applied.

What are tender points? Are they the same as trigger points?

Tender points are the places where the ligaments attach the muscles to bone. Trigger points are spots that will cause pain at another location when pressed. (This is called *referred pain*.) Although the terms were used interchangeably at one time, they are not the same.

What are some of the conditions that can accompany FM?

Not everyone develops all of the following conditions. Some people experience some of them, some of the time. They include: headaches, irritable bowel syndrome, Raynaud's syndrome, painful menstruation, depression, subjective swelling of the hands and feet, a feeling of numbness or tingling in the hands, shortness of breath, a staggering walk upon first arising in the morning, and dryness of the mucous membranes in the nose, mouth, and other locations.

Can a person have fibromyalgia and a form of arthritis?
Yes. Some people with fibromyalgia also have rheumatoid arthritis, osteoarthritis, lupus, or other types of arthritis.

What affects FM?
Generally, the symptoms are made worse by damp, cold weather, sitting in a draft or in front of an air conditioner, stress, overexertion, or inactivity. Warm, dry weather, warm baths, and rest may ease the symptoms.

Who gets FM?
Studies are still being conducted on the demographics of FM, but at this time we do know that more women than men get FM, and generally it affects those between the 30s and 60s. However, it has been found in a few teenagers and in some people in their 70s. It is also a possibility that many adults first experienced FM while teenagers, but were unaware of it at the time.

What causes FM?
At this time, it is not known what causes fibromyalgia. The onset can sometimes be traced to an accident, an emotional trauma, or a viral-like illness. But in other cases, the onset is gradual, making it difficult to know when symptoms first appeared.

Why do I feel so tired?
People with FM often have regular disruptions in their sleep patterns. Studies have shown that the deepest level (stage four) of sleep is often disrupted. It is during this stage of sleep that the body is restored. But for those with FM, this deep sleep is continually disrupted as if there were an alarm constantly going off, preventing the sleeper from awakening refreshed. The symptoms of FM—pain, stiffness, and fatigue—have been reproduced in healthy subjects by continually disturbing their stage-four sleep.

Is fibromyalgia contagious?
No.

Does FM run in the family? Can my children inherit it?
At this point, that is unclear. There have been some cases in which more than one member of a family has had FM, and some studies have shown a possible tendency for it to run in families.

What tests are used to diagnose FM?
At this time, nothing shows up on either lab work or X rays.

Is FM crippling or life-threatening?
No, but the pain and fatigue can become disabling. Everyone's case is different.

Some people experience only minor fatigue and pain, which can be treated with mild analgesics. Others find it difficult to carry on their normal daily activities.

What can I expect in the long run?

Studies have not found FM to be progressive, but it is adversely affected by such factors as stress and extreme physical activity or inactivity. People who have had a few years of treatment still report pain and fatigue. Remissions can and do occur, but, again, that varies with each person. A remission is considered to be at least a two-month period without pain and stiffness. Some remission periods have lasted years.

Is FM the same disease as chronic fatigue syndrome/chronic fatigue immune dysfunction syndrome (CFIDS)?

Some researchers believe that there is a group of patients who meet the criteria for both fibromyalgia and chronic fatigue syndrome.

Can children get FM?

It has been diagnosed in some children, but it is not common.

What kind of doctor should I see for treatment?

Generally, a rheumatologist treats fibromyalgia, but as more and more family physicians and internal medicine physicians learn about FM, they can also treat you.

How can I find a doctor who treats fibromyalgia?

Contact your local chapter of the Arthritis Foundation or Arthritis Society. These organizations normally maintain a list of doctors. If there is no chapter near you, contact your local medical society or hospital for a list of doctors.

What kind of treatment can I expect?

Every person should be treated individually. At this time, tricyclic antidepressants such as Endep and Elavil are commonly prescribed to improve sleep. These are given in much lower dosages than when they are prescribed for depression. Also muscle relaxers like Flexeril, which is also a tricyclic medication, may be prescribed. Sometimes a nonsteroid, anti-inflammatory drug may be prescribed for pain if regular aspirin or acetaminophen (Tylenol) does not work.

What other kinds of treatment can I expect?

Often a doctor will refer you to a physical therapist, who may use heat or cold to relax the muscles. A physical therapist may also use ultrasound treatments and may teach you some exercises that you can do at home.

What can I expect from my doctor?

The first step is to develop a good doctor-patient relationship. This means that you must be willing to take an active part in your care. Your doctor should confirm your diagnosis, provide assurance that the condition is not life threatening or crippling. Treatment for FM can be frustrating for both doctor and patient, and often you will want your doctor to spend some time with you. That is your right as a patient, but remember that your doctor has other patients as well. Do not expect a magic cure. FM is a chronic condition.

What other health care providers should I see?

Your doctor may refer you to a physical therapist, as already mentioned, but you may also want to see an occupational therapist, a social worker, and a psychologist or psychiatrist.

How do I find these health care professionals?

Any of these specialists' services may be available at your local hospital. Even if you have not been hospitalized, you may still use some of these services. Physical therapists, psychologists, and psychiatrists in private practice can also see you. Generally, your doctor will refer you. Even if you have not been hospitalized, you may contact the social worker on staff at a hospital for referrals and assistance with financial and other needs. Occupational therapists may also be affiliated with universities or medical schools that offer an occupational therapy degree program.

What does an occupational therapist do?

The function of an occupational therapist is to find ways to assist you in continuing your activities in your chosen roles. The therapist can evaluate your home and job environment to find ways to help you conserve energy and ease muscle strain. He or she can also help find or develop adaptive devices that will help you continue to function.

What does a social worker do?

A social worker helps people find ways to handle financial and social problems.

What does a psychologist do for a person with FM?

Psychologists provide counseling services to people with FM who are grieving for the loss of their health, who are angry about the changes in their lifestyles, or who are experiencing other emotional problems brought on by a chronic illness. They can also assist family members in coping with the changes FM has caused. Sometimes they also offer stress management, biofeedback, self-hypnosis, or relaxation therapy training.

My doctor believes my symptoms are all in my head. What can I do?

Because of the lack of evidence in either tests or X rays, some doctors still believe fibromyalgia is a psychological problem. There are other doctors who recognize FM as a physiological problem and treat it accordingly. Continue to look until you find a doctor who takes this approach.

How can I learn more about FM?

As more and more research is conducted, more information is becoming available. If there is a medical school library near you, check the listings in *Index Medicus*, which covers most of the medical journals published today. Another source of information is a support group or association that provides such information. Check with the Arthritis Foundation or the Arthritis Society. The Arthritis Foundation publishes a bi-monthly magazine, which is available to anyone who makes a donation of $20 or more. Addresses for the Arthritis Foundation and the Arthritis society chapter offices and for a number of fibromyalgia associations and support groups are listed in the appendix. You may also subscribe to *Fibromyalgia Network*, a quarterly newsletter (see the Appendix).

What is a support group?

A support group is usually a collection of people who share the same interest in a topic, such as fibromyalgia. They work to provide information and emotional support for each other when others outside the group are unable to. They may or may not meet on a regular basis, publish a newsletter, or maintain a library of material on FM.

How do I find a support group?

The appendix lists a number of support groups around the country, but there may be one in your area that isn't included. Contact your doctor, hospital, local medical society, or newspaper to find one. If there is not a group in your area, you might consider organizing one yourself. Contact the California Network of Self-Help Centers, the Canadian Council on Social Development, the Arthritis Foundation, or the Arthritis Society (see the appendix for their addresses) for assistance in starting a self-help group.

Can I donate blood?

The answer is usually yes, but it is best to check with your own physician first.

What research is being done on fibromyalgia?

At this time, more and more physicians and research centers are becoming interested in fibromyalgia. As the search for the cause of FM continues, there seem to be two directions of research. One group believes that the muscle is responsible for the pain. Some changes, which appear to be caused by microtrauma, have been discovered in the muscles of people with FM. The cause of such microtrauma is still uncertain.

Another group believes that the answer lies within the highly sensitized pain perception of the central nervous system.

How can I cope with my pain if I can't use pain pills?

Anytime someone has a chronic pain condition, it is unwise to use narcotic analgesics, or pain pills, because of the danger of developing an addiction. Using these drugs is also problematic because the longer you use them, the more you have to take to provide the same level of relief. There are some alternative methods of dealing with the pain, which include stress management, distraction, relaxation therapy, self-hypnosis, and biofeedback.

What if I can't maintain my level of work or if I can't keep working at my job?

There are several options that you might consider. The first is to attempt to retain your job. You might consider some changes that will make your job easier.

However, not all supervisors and employers are willing to make such changes.

You may need to cut down from full-time work to a part-time job that will put less strain and stress on you. Stress can make FM's symptoms worse. You might become self-employed, so that you can pace yourself according to your FM.

If you have to make a drastic change in your employment situation, you may be eligible for vocational rehabilitation. The appendix lists addresses for each state's vocational rehabilitation services office. Contact your state office to find branch nearest you.

If I can't work, can I draw Social Security Disability?
The Social Security Administration is still having a difficult time handling applicants with fibromyalgia because there no medical tests, exams, or X rays can provide adequate documentation of the syndrome's existence. Each case is assessed individually, but few applicants have been granted disability benefits. Some of this is affected by your age and education.

What do I tell my family and friends about FM?
You might have your family members read this book. For younger members of the family, explain that you have to make some changes in your lifestyle because of FM. They need to know that it is not life threatening, but that there will be days when you are in pain and may not be able to do some of the things you had planned.

As for how much you explain to friends, that depends on how close you are. Some might also be interested in reading this book. But for every friend who wants to learn about FM, there will be an acquaintance who doesn't realize that FM is a chronic condition that fluctuates from day to day.

A Final Word

I hope this book will give you the information you need to live and cope with fibromyalgia. Or, at least, I hope that it has answered your questions and shown you where to turn if you need more help. I invite you to join me in realizing the possibilities for living a quality life—because there is much more than just surviving FM.

APPENDIX

Health Care Professionals Who Can Help

Counselors and psychologists provide psychological and emotional support and guidance while helping people and their families cope with chronic illness, depression, and stress. They may be affiliated with a medical facility, have a private practice, or work with a local human services agency.

Dietitians/nutritionists provide assistance on special dietary or nutritional needs and food preparation.

Family physicians have advanced training in family medicine and provide medical care for adults and children. When needed, they can refer patients to specialists.

Internists have advanced training in internal medicine and in caring for diseases in adults. They can also refer their patients to specialists.

Nurses work in many environments, from the hospital to doctors' offices and private homes. They can assist your doctor in providing you with health care.

Occupational therapists are registered practitioners who also require a referral from your doctor. They work to help you conserve energy and ease strain on muscles as you fulfill the day-to-day activities that your various roles require. They can evaluate your work and home environments and suggest ways you can function more easily in those environments.

Pharmacists fill your doctor's prescriptions and can provide information about a drug's side effects and the way it responds when mixed with other medications. They can also advise you about over-the-counter medications.

Physiatrists are doctors who specialize in rehabilitation and treat symptoms with the help of such agents as heat, cold, water, electricity, and mechanical apparatus.

Physical therapists are licensed practitioners who work with you on your physician's orders. They can teach you exercises that will help maintain muscle strength and provide relief without using medication for pain control.

Psychiatrists are physicians who treat and prevent mental disorders. Unlike psychologists, psychiatrists can prescribe medication for such problems.

Rheumatologists specialize in the treatment of arthritis and rheumatic diseases.

Social workers can be affiliated with hospitals or medical centers, where they work to help people handle financial and social problems. They may provide counseling or assistance in learning coping skills.

Vocational rehabilitation counselors have special training to help those with physical or mental handicaps retain their jobs, obtain work, or reenter the work force.

Note: Not everyone will require the services of all the health care providers listed.

Arthritis Foundation Chapters

ALABAMA

Alabama Chapter
200 Vestavia Parkway
Suite 3050
Birmingham, Alabama 35216
(205) 979-5700

South Alabama Chapter
1720 Springhill Avenue
Mobile, Alabama 36604
(205) 432-7171

ALASKA

Alaska Unit
c/o Arthritis Foundation
1314 Spring Street, NW
Atlanta, Georgia 30309
(404) 872-7100

ARIZONA

Central Arizona Chapter
711 East Missouri Avenue
Suite 116
Phoenix, Arizona 85014
(602) 264-7679

Southern Arizona Chapter
6464 East Grant Road
Tucson, Arizona 85715
(602) 290-9090

ARKANSAS

Arkansas Chapter
6213 Lee Avenue
Little Rock, Arkansas 72205
(501) 664-7242

CALIFORNIA

Northeastern California Chapter
2424 Arden Way
Suite 450
Sacramento, California 95825
(916) 921-5533

Northern California Chapter
203 Willow Street
Suite 201
San Francisco, California 94109
(415) 673-6882

San Diego Chapter
7675 Dagget Street
Suite 330
San Diego, California 92111-2241
(619) 492-1094

Southern California Chapter
4311 Wilshire Boulevard
Suite 530
Los Angeles, California 90010
(213) 938-6111

COLORADO
Rocky Mountain Chapter
2280 South Albion Street
Denver, Colorado 80222
(303) 756-8622

CONNECTICUT
Connecticut Chapter
1092 Elm Street
Rocky Hill, Connecticut 06067
(203) 563-1177

DELAWARE
Delaware Chapter
222 Philadelphia Pike, #1
Wilmington, Delaware 19809
(302) 764-8254

DISTRICT OF COLUMBIA
Metro Washington Chapter
1901 Ft. Myer Drive
Suite 500
Arlington, Virginia 22209
(703) 276-7555

FLORIDA
Florida Chapter
5211 Manatee Avenue, West
Bradenton, Florida 34209
(813) 795-3010

GEORGIA
Georgia Chapter
2045 Peachtree Road, NE, #800
Atlanta, Georgia 30309-1405
(404) 351-0454

HAWAII
Hawaii Chapter
Honfed Bank Building
45-1144 Kamehameha Highway
Kaneohe, Hawaii 96744
(808) 235-3636

IDAHO
Idaho Chapter
4696 Overland Road
Suite 538
Boise, Idaho 83705
(208) 344-7102

ILLINOIS
Central Illinois Chapter
2621 North Knoxville
Peoria, Illinois 61604
(309) 682-6600

Illinois Chapter
79 West Monroe Street
Suite 510
Chicago, Illinois 60603
(312) 782-1367

INDIANA
Indiana Chapter
8646 Guion Road
Indianapolis, Indiana 46268-3011
(317) 879-0321

IOWA
Iowa Chapter
8410 Hickman
Suite A
Des Moines, Iowa 50325
(515) 278-0636

KANSAS
Kansas Chapter
1602 East Waterman
Wichita, Kansas 67211
(316) 263-0116

KENTUCKY
Kentucky Chapter
3900B DuPont Square South
Louisville, Kentucky 40207-4615
(502) 893-9771

LOUISIANA
Louisiana Chapter
3955 Government Street
Suite 7
Baton Rouge, Louisiana 70806
(504) 387-6932

MAINE
Maine Chapter
37 Mill Street
Brunswick, Maine 04011
(207) 729-4453

MARYLAND
Maryland Chapter
3 Lan Lea Drive
Lutherville, Maryland 21093
(301) 561-8090

MASSACHUSETTS
Massachusetts Chapter
29 Crafts Street
450 Chatham Center
Newton, Massachusetts 02160
(617) 244-1800

MICHIGAN
Michigan Chapter
23999 Northwestern Highway
Suite 210
Southfield, Michigan 48075
(313) 350-3030

MINNESOTA
Minnesota Chapter
1730 Clifton Place
Suite AI
Minneapolis, Minnesota 55403
(612) 874-9332

MISSISSIPPI
Mississippi Chapter
6055 Ridgewood Road
Jackson, Mississippi 39211
(601) 956-3371

MISSOURI
Eastern Missouri Chapter
7315 Manchester
St. Louis, Missouri 63143
(314) 644-3488

Western Missouri/Greater Kansas
  City Chapter
8301 State Line
Suite 200
Kansas City, Missouri 64114
(816) 361-7002

MONTANA
Montana Chapter
c/o Arthritis Foundation
1314 Spring Street
Atlanta, Georgia 30309
(404) 872-7100

NEBRASKA
Nebraska Chapter
2229 North 91st Court
Suite 33
Omaha, Nebraska 68134
(402) 391-8000

NEVADA
Nevada Chapter
3850 West Desert Inn Road
Suite 108
Las Vegas, Nevada 89102
(702) 367-1626

NEW HAMPSHIRE
New Hampshire Chapter
$2^{1}/_{2}$ Beacon Street, #10
Concord, New Hampshire 03301
(603) 224-9322

NEW JERSEY
New Jersey Chapter
200 Middlesex Turnpike
Iselin, New Jersey 08830
(908) 283-4300

NEW MEXICO
New Mexico Chapter
124 Alvarado, Southeast
P.O. Box 8022
Albuquerque, New Mexico 87108
(505) 265-1545

NEW YORK
Central New York Chapter
The Pickard Building
5858 East Molloy Road
Suite 123
Syracuse, New York 13211
(315) 455-8553

Genesee Valley Chapter
One Mount Hope Road
Rochester, New York 14620-1088
(716) 423-9490

Long Island Chapter
501 Walt Whitman Road
Melville, New York 11747
(516) 427-8272

New York Chapter
67 Irving Place
New York, New York 10003
(212) 477-8310

Northeastern New York Chapter
1717 Central Avenue
Suite 105
Albany, New York 12205
(518) 456-1203

Western New York Chapter
1370 Niagara Falls Boulevard
Tonawanda, New York 14150
(716) 837-8600

NORTH CAROLINA
North Carolina Chapter
3801 Wake Forest Road, #115
Durham, North Carolina 27703
(919) 596-3360

NORTH DAKOTA
Dakota Chapter
115 Roberts Street
Fargo, North Dakota 58102
(701) 237-3310

OHIO
Central Ohio Chapter
2501 North Star Road
Columbus, Ohio 43221
(614) 488-0777

Northeastern Ohio Chapter
23811 Chagrin Boulevard
Chagrin Plaza East
Suite 210
Beachwood, Ohio 44122
(216) 831-7000

Northwestern Ohio Chapter
2650 North Reynolds Road
Toledo, Ohio 43615
(419) 537-0888

Southwestern Ohio Chapter
7811 Laurel Avenue
Cincinnati, Ohio 45243
(513) 271-4545

OKLAHOMA
Eastern Oklahoma Chapter
4520 West Harvard, #100
Tulsa, Oklahoma 74135
(918) 743-4526

Oklahoma Chapter
2915 Classen Boulevard, #325
Oklahoma City, Oklahoma
    73106-5466
(405) 521-0066

OREGON
Oregon Chapter
4412 Southwest Barbur Boulevard
Suite 220
Portland, Oregon 97201
(503) 222-7246

PENNSYLVANIA
Central Pennsylvania Chapter
17 South 19th Street
P.O. Box 668
Camp HIll, Pennsylvania 17011
(717) 763-0900

Eastern Pennsylvania Chapter
1217 Sansom Street
Philadelphia, Pennsylvania 19107
(215) 574-9480

Western Pennsylvania Chapter
332 Fifth Avenue
Warner Centre, Fifth Floor
Pittsburgh Pennsylvania 15222
(412) 566-1645

RHODE ISLAND
Rhode Island Chapter
850 Waterman Avenue
East Providence, Rhode Island
   02914
(401) 434-5792

SOUTH CAROLINA
South Carolina Chapter
P.O. Box 11967
Columbia, South Carolina
   29202-1967
(803) 254-6702

TENNESSEE
Middle-East Tennessee Chapter
210 25th Avenue North
Suite 523
Nashville, Tennessee 37203
(615) 329-3431

West Tennessee Chapter
6084 Apple Tree Drive
Suite 4
Memphis, Tennessee 38115
(901) 365-7080

TEXAS
North Texas Chapter
2824 Swiss Avenue
Dallas, Texas 75204
(214) 826-4361

Northwest Texas Chapter
3145 McCart Avenue
Fort Worth, Texas 76110
(817) 926-7733

South Central Texas Chapter
1407 North Main
San Antonio, Texas 78212
(512) 224-8222

Texas Gulf Coast Chapter
7660 Woodway
Suite 540
Houston, Texas 77063
(713) 785-2360

UTAH
Utah Chapter
1733 South 1100 East
Salt Lake City, Utah 84105
(801) 486-4993

VERMONT
Vermont & Northern New York
   Chapter
P.O. Box 422
Burlington, Vermont 05402
(802) 864-4988

VIRGINIA
Virginia Chapter
565 Southlake Boulevard
Richmond, Virginia 23236
(804) 379-7464

WASHINGTON
Washington State Chapter
100 South King, #330
Seattle, Washington 98104
(206) 622-1378

WEST VIRGINIA
West Virginia Chapter
2307 Chapline Street
Wheeling, West Virginia 26003
(304) 232-5810

WISCONSIN
Wisconsin Chapter
8556 West National Avenue
West Allis, Wisconsin 53227
(414) 321-3933

NATIONAL HEADQUARTERS
1314 Spring Street, Northwest
Atlanta, Georgia 30309
(404) 872-7100

*Contact your state chapter office for information on the branch office nearest you.

The Arthritis Society of Canada

National Office
250 Bloor Street East
Suite 401
Toronto, Ontario M4W 3P2

Newfoundland
Box 522, Station C
St. John's, Newfoundland
    A1C 5K4

Prince Edward Island
P.O. Box 1537
Charlottetown, P.E,I, C1A 7N3

Nova Scotia
5516 Spring Garden Road
Halifax, Nova Scotia B3J 1G6

New Brunswick
65 Brunswick Street
Fredericton, New Brunswick
    E3B 1G5

Quebec
2075 University Street
Suite 1206
Montreal, Quebec H3A 2L1

Ontario
250 Bloor Street East
Suite 401
Toronto, Ontario M4W 3P2

Manitoba
386 Broadway Avenue
Suite 105
Winnipeg, Manitoba R3C 3R6

Saskatchewan
2078 Halifax
Regina, Saskatchewan S4N 0P2

Alberta
301, 1301—8th Street Southwest
Calgary, Alberta T2R 1B7

British Columbia and Yukon
895 West 10th Avenue
Vancouver, British Columbia
    V5Z 1L7

Other Helpful Resources

American College of Rheumatology
17 Executive Park Drive, Northeast
Suite 480
Atlanta, Georgia 30329
(404) 633-3777
A national organization of clinicians and scientists who are exploring new possibilities in the treatment of and cure for the rheumatic diseases. Check membership roster for specialists in your area.

Multipurpose Arthritis Centers (MAC)
A bulletin from the Arthritis Foundation can tell you where these clinical and research centers are currently operating. They are usually located within a university medical center. They provide a variety of services, which differ from center to center, but all perform basic and clinical research; provide professional, patient, and public education; and sponsor community activities.

American Association of Retired Persons
National Headquarters
1909 K Street, Northwest
Washington, D.C. 20049
Provides programs and services to keep members informed about legal, financial, health, and consumer issues. Includes a pharmacy service that provides health and self-help aids at a low cost. Publications include a news bulletin and *Modern Maturity*, a bi-monthly magazine. For those planning retirement, a special division called Action for Independent Maturity produces a magazine, *Dynamic Maturity*, and runs its own programs.

American Occupational Therapy Association
1383 Piccard Drive
Rockville, Maryland 20850
(301) 948-9626
This association can help you locate an occupational therapist in your area and can also direct your search

for information about self-help devices. It offers many publications on occupational therapy.

American Physical Therapy Association

1111 North Fairfax Street
Alexandria, Virginia 22314
(703) 684-2782
This organization can help you locate a physical therapist in your area.

American National Red Cross

17th and D Streets, Northwest
Washington, D.C. 20006
Local chapters run various programs across the country, including home nursing, community service, and youth activity programs. Some chapters loan out equipment and provide transportation and other assistance services.

Amtrak, National Railroad Corporation

400 North Capitol Street,
   Northwest
Washington, D.C. 20001
(202) 383-3000
Publishes *Access Amtrak*, about services for elderly and handicapped travelers, with information on discount fares.

Consumer Information Center

Pueblo, Colorado 81009
Assists federal agencies in developing and releasing relevant, useful consumer information. Also works to increase public awareness on this information. Publishes the *Consumer Information Catalog*, which lists more than 200 federal publica-

tions on topics such as careers, health, nutrition, education, and money management.

Family Service Association of America

44 East 23rd Street
New York, New York 10010
A national accrediting federation for all the local agencies listed under Family Services in the telephone directory. These offices provide counseling and support services including assistance in securing funds you may be entitled to. Funds studies and aims to improve conditions affecting families.

Higher Education and the Handicapped (Health) Resource Center

One Dupont Circle, Northwest
Suite 670
Washington, D.C. 20036-1193
(202) 833-4707
Operates a national clearinghouse on post-secondary education for handicapped people. Information about educational support services, policies, procedures, adaptations, and opportunities on American campuses, vocational-technical schools, adult education programs, independent living centers, and other training after high school. A list of helpful publications is also available.

Small Business Administration (SBA)

Handicapped Assistance Loans (HAL-2) are available to finance a small business owned by a handicapped person. Detailed information can be obtained from the SBA office in your area.

Clearinghouse for the Handicapped

Office of Special Education and
    Rehabilitative Services
United States Department of
    Education
330 C Street, Southwest
Room 3132, Switzer Building
Washington, D.C. 20202
(202) 732-1244

Provides information and referrals for federal and private services for the handicapped. Provides information on recent research developments for the handicapped. Publications include *Directory of National Information Sources on Handicapping Conditions and Related Services* from the Government Printing Office, and *Pocket Guide to Federal Help for the Disabled.*

Disabled Person in the Workplace: An Introductory Reference and Resource Guide

Electronics Industries Foundation
Project with Industry
2001 Eye Street, Northwest
Washington, D.C. 20006

Includes annotated bibliography of publications on accommodation aids, attitudes, devices, employment, equipment, evaluation, and services relevant to the disabled.

Also includes a list of organizations that offer a variety of services to disabled people and their employers.

Job Accommodation Network

P.O. Box 468
Morgantown, West Virginia 26505
(800) 526-7234
(800) 526-4698, West Virginia
    residents

Free nationwide information network and consulting service, providing information on possible accommodations that employers might use so they can hire, retain, or promote disabled people.

National Institute of Arthritis and Musculoskeletal and Skin Diseases Information Clearinghouse

P.O. Box 9782
Arlington, Virginia 22209
(703) 558-8250

Provides information in the areas of patient education, public education, professional education, community demonstration programs, and federal problems on the rheumatic diseases. Write or call for an order form listing materials available by subject.

Office on the Americans With Disabilities Act

Civil Rights Division
United States Department of
    Justice
P.O. Box 66118
Washington, D.C. 20035-6118
(202) 514-0301

Organizations that Help People Who Have Fibromyalgia

The following is a list of organizations that are dedicated to helping those with fibromyalgia, chronic fatigue syndrome, and chronic pain and illness. The next group includes support groups. Although this is the most complete list available, it does not include every group in the United States and Canada. If there is no group in your area on the list, and you cannot find one on your own, consider starting your own. Help for starting such groups can be obtained from any of the following addresses or from the Arthritis Foundation.

The Fibromyalgia Association of Central Ohio
Riverside Hospital
Suite 8
3545 Olentangy River Road
Columbus, Ohio 43214
(614) 262-2000

The Fibromyalgia Association of Texas, Inc.
5650 Forest Lane
Dallas, Texas 75230
(214) 363-2473

Essex County Fibrositis Group
380 Pelissier Street, #1904
Windsor, Ontario N9A 6V7
Canada
(519) 254-5343

Fibromyalgia Association of BC
Box 15455
Vancouver, B.C. V6B 5B2
Canada
(604) 688-0503

Ontario Fibrositis Association
250 Bloor Street East
Suite 401
Toronto, Ontario M4W 3P2
Canada
(416) 967-1414

American Chronic Pain Association
P.O. Box 850
Rocklin, California 95677
(916) 632-0922
Call for local chapters.

**Chronic Fatigue Immune
Dysfunction Syndrome**
(CFIDS) Association
P.O. Box 220398
Charlotte, North Carolina 28222
(800) 442-3437

National Self-Help Clearinghouse
25 West 43rd Street
Room 620
New York, New York 10036

**California Network of Self-Help
Centers**
Attn: Diane Wright, Region III
Merced County Department of
    Mental Health
650 West 19th Street
Merced, California 95340
(209) 385-6937
Offers a free self-help-group starter
packet titled *Helping You Helps Me*.

**Canadian Council on Social
Development**
55 Parkdale Avenue
Ottawa, Ontario K1Y 4G1
Canada
Offers a booklet on how to develop
self-help groups

Fibromyalgia Network Support Groups

ALABAMA
F.A.C.T.
4500 Brentwood Drive
Mobile, Alabama 36619
(205) 661-0344

ARIZONA
Tom Cadden
2115 West Royal Palm, #2027
Phoenix, Arizona 85021
(602) 995-2907

Mrs. Susan Tripoli
3735 North Tanuri Drive
Tucson, Arizona 85715
(602) 885-8992

ARKANSAS
Mary Alice Beer
Route 3, Box 51-D
Fairfield, Arkansas 72088
(501) 884-3502

CALIFORNIA
Jane Meyer
1115 19th Street, #8
Santa Monica, California 90403
(213) 828-6536

Diane Isaacs
P.O. Box 554
La Canada, California 91012
(818) 790-1420

Lois Merrill
742 Baylor Avenue
Chula Vista, California 92010
(619) 421-8908

Carolyn Hendrickson
11222 Culver Court
El Cajon, California 92020
(619) 442-2423

Rosalie McKinley
2141 Oro Verde Road
Escondido, California 92027
(619) 745-2862

Renee Bradbury
56105 Pueblo Trail
Yucca Valley, California 92284
(619) 365-5073

Pat Atwell
1524A Brookhollow
Santa Ana, California 92705
(714) 668-1623

Iona Cridland
810 South Clementine
Anaheim, California 92805
(714) 774-1255

Anna Bermudez
601 Eva Street
Ventura, California 93003
(805) 644-3583

Karen Duren
16441 Grant Line Road
Tracy, California 95376
(415) 447-2393

Bernita Creech
2721 13th Street
Sacramento, California 95818
(916) 446-0918

COLORADO
Shelli Dimig
4735 East 129th Court
Thornton, Colorado 80241
(303) 452-1052

Lonnie B. Grove
P.O. Box 46
Atwood, Colorado 80722
(303) 522-1045

CONNECTICUT
Margaret Ann Moi
29 Jefferson Street
Unionville, Connecticut 06085
(203) 673-1913

FLORIDA
Carolyn Bell
P.O. Box 5491
Gainesville, Florida 32602
(904) 964-5847

Joan Wackerly
4727 Northwest 19th Place
Gainesville, Florida 32605
(904) 373-6865

Howard Aaron
231 174th Street, #312
Miami, Florida 33160-3315
(305) 935-5657

Betty Rohde
3910 Sunnybrook Lane
Lakeland, Florida 33801
(813) 683-1447

Loretta Gotsch
P.O. Box 285
517 Main Street
Lake Hamilton, Florida 33851
(813) 439-1149

Cathie McIntyre
3206 Ramblewood Drive, North
Sarasota, Florida 34237
(813) 955-5831

Jackie Dunnington
24 Maplewood Avenue
Clearwater, Florida 34625-3330
(813) 797-2360

Becky Frase
202 East Dartmouth
Oldsmar, Florida 34677
(813) 855-7765

GEORGIA
Arthritis Care Center
2701 North Decatur Road
Decatur, Georgia 30033
(404) 501-2784

Lorraine Dress, R.P.T.
5444 Chanterella Court
Lilburn, Georgia 30247
(404) 501-2784

Atlanta CFS Association
P.O. Box 29891
Atlanta, Georgia 30359
(404) 662-6819

ILLINOIS
Kathy Henderson
26 West 110 Durfee Road
Wheaton, Illinois 60187
(708) 260-0323

Becky Heiman
28 Bayshore Drive
Lacon, Illinois 61540
(309) 246-8963

Joyce Moncelle-Kaye
1016 East Washington Street
Bloomington, Illinois 61701
(309) 828-3936

INDIANA
Indiana CFS Support Group
810 North Bancroft
Indianapolis, Indiana 46201
(317) 252-9223

LOUISIANA
Charlotte Lawson
1331 Beckenham Drive
Baton Rouge, Louisiana 70808
(504) 769-7286

MAINE
Central Maine CFIDS Association
RD2, Box 525
Manchester, Maine 04351
(207) 395-4464

MARYLAND
Jan Thompson
22 Truckhouse Road
Severna Park, Maryland 21146
(301) 544-5433

MASSACHUSETTS
Massachusetts CFIDS Association
808 Main Street
Waltham, Massachusetts 02154
(617) 893-4415

Lorraine Forman
84 Pond Lane
Randolph, Maine 02368
(617) 963-2507

MINNESOTA
Rosalie Devonshire
460 Highcroft Road
Wayzata, Minnesota 55391
(612) 476-7323

MISSOURI
Lona Polk
1209 West 9th Street
Washington, Missouri 63090
(314) 239-0273

NEW HAMPSHIRE
Linda Boehme
RFD #1, Box 79
Andover, New Hampshire 03216
(603) 735-5384

NEW JERSEY
Grace C. Cerrato
274 Riva Drive
Hackettstown, New Jersey 07840
(908) 850-8695

Lila Roseman
13 Bennington Court
East Brunswick, New Jersey
   08816
(908) 283-4300

NEW MEXICO
Sue Alice Erickson, C.H.E.S.
2904 Calle Grande Northwest
Albuquerque, New Mexico 87104
(505) 344-2640

Dennis Reublin
1009 Rocky Point Court, Northeast
Albuquerque, New Mexico 87123
(505) 296-1358

NEW YORK
Patricia Olive
30 Pierrepoint Street
Brooklyn, New York 11201
(718) 624-2955

Sheila Moceyunas
111 Washington Boulevard
Fayetteville, New York 13066
(315) 637-8054

NORTH CAROLINA
Cindy Berrier, R.N.
1945 Randolph Road
Charlotte, North Carolina 28207
(704) 331-4878

OHIO
Ruth Buzard, R.N.
3545 Olentangy River, Road, #8
Columbus, Ohio 43214
(614) 451-9532

Patricia Beede
5385 Market Street
Youngstown, Ohio 44512
(216) 782-6302

Lisa McCormick
2141 Auburn Avenue
Cincinnati, Ohio 45219
(513) 369-2737

OKLAHOMA
Kathy Burris
10061 South Sheridan Road, #615
Tulsa, Oklahoma 74133
(918) 299-1939

PENNSYLVANIA
Patricia Youngren
P.O. Box 122
Jennerstown, Pennsylvania 15547
(814) 629-9093

Shirley Thompson
P.O. Box 156
Freeport, Pennsylvania 16229
(412) 295-2777

Alice Kurceba
319 Simms Street
Suite 101
Philadelphia, Pennsylvania 19116
(215) 464-6369

RHODE ISLAND
Pat Dugas
29 Watercress Court
Coventry, Rhode Island 02816
(401) 828-5354

Debbie Burgess
18 Newwood Drive
Cranston, Rhode Island 02920
(401) 463-8305

SOUTH CAROLINA
Sally Reid
119 Wilshire Drive
Greenville, South Carolina 29609
(803) 233-8815

Oconee County CFIDS Group
P.O. Box 114
Mountain Rest, South Carolina
  29664
(803) 638-7615

TEXAS
Karen Samuelsohn
5650 Forest Lane
Dallas, Texas 75230
(214) 363-2473

Joan Reilly-Bertsch
7539 Alverstone Way
San Antonio, Texas 78250
(512) 522-9410

Genevieve Williams
3312 88th Street
Lubbock, Texas 79423
(806) 745-7328

Gayle Backstrom
2212 Fort Worth Drive, #94
Denton, Texas 76205
(817) 382-0415

UTAH
Barbara Nebeker
3227 Plum Tree Lane
Bountiful, Utah 84010
(801) 295-1916

Lujean Anderson
4562 North 50 West
Provo, Utah 84604
(801) 226-7686

VIRGINIA
Lan LeBosquet
P.O. Box 83
Dunn Loring, Virginia 22027
(703) 560-9408

WASHINGTON
Patricia Hendricksen
5507 Kenwood Place North, #204
Seattle, Washington 98103
(206) 634-2275

Joan Harris
East 9711 Maringo Drive
Spokane, Washington 99206
(509) 926-8683

WEST VIRGINIA
Meadowbrook CFIDS Group
Rt. 3, Box 35
Salem, West Virginia 26426
(304) 782-3372

WISCONSIN
Ingrid Regal
13675 West Burleigh Road
Brookfield, Wisconsin 53005
(414) 782-0346

CANADA
Lynda Snow
100 Downsview Drive
Saint John, New Brunswick
    E2M 5E3
(506) 674-1156

Diane H. Clarke
186 Beaconsfield Street
Fredericton, New Brunswick
    E3B 5H2
(506) 459-0261

Joan Kenny
68 Elgin Street
Fredericton, New Brunswick
    E3B 5P9
(506) 452-7677

Melba Halfpenny
5475 Lakeshore Road
Burlington, Ontario L7L 1E1
(416) 967-1414

Joan A. Brown
1904–380 Pelissier Street
Windsor, Ontario N9A 6V7
(519) 254-5343

Beverley Fujino, CFS Director
Box 30402
1323N–6455 MacLeod TrSW
Calgary, Alberta T2H 2W2
(403) 243-3169

Mrs. Joan Greene
3344 10th Avenue
Mission, British Columbia V2V
   2K6
(604) 826-6070

Anna Abel
4917–197 A Street
Langley, British Columbia V3A
   6W1
(604) 534-8400

Judy Verstick
1250 Bute Street, #1203
Vancouver, British Columbia V6E
   1Z9
(604) 688-0503

State Vocational Rehabilitation Offices

Call the following state offices for the office nearest you.

ALABAMA
Division of Rehabilitation Services
P.O. Box 11586
2129 East South Boulevard
Montgomery, Alabama
  36111-0586
(205) 281-8780

ALASKA
Division of Vocational
  Rehabilitation
P.O. Box F
Mail Stop 0581
Juneau, Alaska 99811-0500
(907) 465-2814

ARIZONA
Rehabilitation Services
  Administration
Department of Economic Security
1300 West Washington Street,
  930A
Phoenix, Arizona 85007
(602) 542-3332

ARKANSAS
Division of Rehabilitation Services
Department of Human Services
P.O. Box 3781
Little Rock, Arkansas 72203
(501) 682-6697

CALIFORNIA
Department of Rehabilitation
830 K Street Mall
Sacramento, California 95814
(916) 445-3971

COLORADO
Rehabilitation Services
1575 Sherman Street, 4th Floor
Denver, Colorado 80203
(303) 866-4390

CONNECTICUT
Department of Human Resources
Bureau of Rehabilitation Services
10 Griffin Road, North
Windsor, Connecticut 06095
(203) 298-2003

DELAWARE
Division of Vocational
   Rehabilitation
Delaware Elwyn Institutes
   4th Floor
321 East 11th Street
Wilmington, Delaware 19801
(302) 577-2850

DISTRICT OF COLUMBIA
D.C. Rehabilitation Services
Commission on Social Services
Department of Human Services
605 G Street, Northwest
   Room 1101
Washington, D.C. 20001
(202) 727-3227

FLORIDA
Division of Vocational
   Rehabilitation
Department of Labor and
   Employment Security
1709A Mahan Drive
Tallahassee, Florida 32399-0696
(904) 488-6210

GEORGIA
Division of Rehabilitation
Department of Human Services
878 Peachtree Street, Northeast
Room 706
Atlanta, Georgia 30309
(404) 894-6670

HAWAII
Division of Vocational
   Rehabilitation
Department of Human Services
P.O. Box 339
1000 Bishop Street
Suite 605
Honolulu, Hawaii 96809
(808) 586-5355

IDAHO
Division of Vocational
   Rehabilitation
Len B. Jordon Building, Room 150
650 West State
Boise, Idaho 83720
(208) 334-3390

ILLINOIS
Department of Rehabilitation
   Services
623 East Adams Street
P.O. Box 19429
Springfield, Illinois 62794-9429
(217) 782-2093

INDIANA
Department of Human Services
P.O. Box 7083
402 West Washington Street
Suite C451
Indianapolis, Indiana 46207-7083
(317) 232-1139

IOWA
Division of Vocational
   Rehabilitation Services
Department of Education
510 East 12th Street
Des Moines, Iowa 50319
(515) 281-4311

KANSAS
Division of Rehabilitation Services
300 Southwest Oakley
Biddle Building, 1st Floor
Topeka, Kansas 66606
(913) 296-3911

KENTUCKY
Department of Vocational
   Rehabilitation
Bureau of Rehabilitative Services
Capital Plaza Office Tower
   9th Floor
Frankfort, Kentucky 40601
(502) 564-4566

LOUISIANA
Division of Rehabilitation Services
Office of Community Services
P.O. Box 94371
1755 Florida
Baton Rouge, Louisiana 70821
(504) 342-2285

MAINE
Bureau of Rehabilitation
Department of Human Services
35 Anthony Avenue
Augusta, Maine 04333
(207) 289-2266

MARYLAND
Division of Vocational
   Rehabilitation
State Department of Education
2301 Argonne Drive
Baltimore, Maryland 21218
(301) 554-3276

MASSACHUSETTS
Rehabilitation Commission
27–43 Wormwood Street, 6th
   Floor
Boston, Massachusetts 02110
(617) 727-2172

MICHIGAN
Michigan Rehabilitation Services
P.O. Box 30010
608 West Allegan Street
Lansing, Michigan 48909
(517) 373-3391

MINNESOTA
Division of Rehabilitation Services
390 North Robert Street, 5th Floor
St. Paul, Minnesota 55101
(612) 296-5616

MISSISSIPPI
Vocational Rehabilitation Services
P.O. Box 1698
932 North State Street
Jackson, Mississippi 39215-1698
(601) 354-6825

MISSOURI
State Department of Education
Division of Vocational
   Rehabilitation
2401 East McCarty
Jefferson City, Missouri 65101
(314) 751-3251

MONTANA
Department of Social and
   Rehabilitation Services
Rehabilitative Services Division
P.O. Box 4210
111 Sanders
Helena, Montana 59604
(406) 444-2590

NEBRASKA
Division of Rehabilitation Service
State Department of Education
301 Centennial Mall, South
6th Floor
P.O. 94987
Lincoln, Nebraska 68509
(402) 471-3652

NEVADA
Department of Human Resources
   Rehabilitation Division
505 East King Street, Room 502
Carson City, Nevada 89710
(702) 687-4440

NEW HAMPSHIRE
Division of Vocational
    Rehabilitation
State Department of Education
78 Regional Drive, Building JB
Concord, New Hampshire 03301
(603) 271-3471

NEW JERSEY
Division of Vocational
    Rehabilitation Services
Department of Labor and Industry
John Fitch Plaza, Room 612
Trenton, New Jersey 08625
(609) 292-5987

NEW MEXICO
Division of Vocational
    Rehabilitation
State Department of Education
604 West San Mateo
Santa Fe, New Mexico 87503
(505) 827-3511

NEW YORK
Office of Vocational and
    Educational Services for
    Individuals with Disabilities
Room 1606
99 Washington Avenue
Albany, New York 12234
(518) 474-2714

NORTH CAROLINA
Division of Vocational
    Rehabilitation Services
Department of Human Resources
P.O. Box 26053
805 Ruggles Drive
Raleigh, North Carolina 27611
(919) 733-3364

NORTH DAKOTA
Office of Vocational Rehabilitation
Department of Human Services
400 Broadway, Room 303
Bismarck, North Dakota
    58501-4038
(701) 224-9999

OHIO
Ohio Rehabilitation Services
    Commission
400 East Campus View Boulevard
Columbus, Ohio 43235-4604
(614) 438-1210

OKLAHOMA
Division of Rehabilitation
Department of Human Resources
2409 North Kelly, Annex Building
P.O. Box 25352
Oklahoma City, Oklahoma 73125
(405) 424-4311

OREGON
Division of Vocational
    Rehabilitation
Department of Human Services
2045 Silverton Road, Northeast
Salem, Oregon 97310
(503) 378-3850

PENNSYLVANIA
Office of Vocational Rehabilitation
Labor and Industry Building
7th and Forster Streets
Harrisburg, Pennsylvania 17120
(717) 787-5244

RHODE ISLAND
Vocational Rehabilitation
Department of Human Services
40 Fountain Street
Providence, Rhode Island 02903
(401) 421-7005

SOUTH CAROLINA
Vocational Rehabilitation
Department
P.O. Box 15
1410 Boston Avenue
West Columbia, South Carolina
29171-0015
(803) 734-4300

SOUTH DAKOTA
Division of Vocational
Rehabilitation
700 Governors Drive
Pierre, South Dakota 57501
(605) 773-3195

TENNESSEE
Division of Rehabilitation Services
Department of Human Services
Citizens Plaza
State Office Building,
15th Floor
400 Deaderick Street
Nashville, Tennessee 37248-6000
(615) 741-2030

TEXAS
Rehabilitation Commission
118 East Riverside Drive
Austin, Texas 78704
(512) 445-8108

UTAH
Office of Rehabilitation
250 East 5th South
Salt Lake City, Utah 84111
(801) 538-7530

VERMONT
Vocational Rehabilitation Division
Agency of Human Services
Osgood Building, Waterbury
Complex
103 South Main Street
Waterbury, Vermont 05671-2303
(802) 241-2189

VIRGINIA
Department of Rehabilitative
Services
Commonwealth of Virginia
4901 Fitzhugh Avenue
P.O. Box 11045
Richmond, Virginia 23230
(804) 367-1641

WASHINGTON
Division of Vocational
Rehabilitation
Department of Social and Health
Services
OB 21 C
Olympia, Washington 98504
(206) 753-2544

WEST VIRGINIA
Division of Rehabilitation Services
State Capitol
Charleston, West Virginia 25305
(304) 766-4601

WISCONSIN
Division of Vocational
Rehabilitation
Department of Health and Social
Services
1 West Wilson, 8th Floor
P.O. Box 7852
Madison, Wisconsin 53707
(608) 266-2168

WYOMING
Division of Vocational
    Rehabilitation
Department of Health and
    Employment
1100 Herschler Building
Cheyenne, Wyoming 82002
(307) 777-7385

Special Publications

Fibromyalgia Network

A quarterly newsletter devoted to fibromyalgia/fibrositis/CFIDS-related topics. $15 per year in the United States, $17 per year in Canada, and $20 per year outside of North America. Write Fibromyalgia Network, 5700 Stockdale Hwy., Suite 100, Bakersfield, California 93309-2768.

The six most recent back issues are available for $15 in the United States, $17 in Canada, and $20 outside of North America.

The Fibromyalgia Network is devoted to providing patients and health care professionals with up-to-date information on fibromyalgia research, new medications, and suggestions for coping with the unyielding symptoms of this chronic condition. News on chronic fatigue immune dysfunction syndrome (CFIDS) is also included.

Accent on Living
Accent Publications
P.O. Box 700
Bloomington, Illinois 61702-0700
Lists new helpful products and services.

American Rehabilitation
U.S. Government Printing Office
Superintendent of Documents
Washington, D.C. 20402
Covers all aspects of rehabilitation, with emphasis on vocational training and independent living.

Arthritis Today
Arthritis Foundation
1314 Spring Street, Northwest
Atlanta, Georgia 30309

Information on Medicare and Health Insurance
American Association of Retired Persons
Fulfillment Section
P.O. Box 2400
Long Beach, California 90801
This free booklet explains what Medicare does and does not cover and describes various additional types of insurance.

Pocket Guide to Federal Help for the Disabled Person
Clearinghouse on the Handicapped
Office of Special Education and Rehabilitation Services
330 C Street, Southwest

(Cont.)

Office of Special Education and Rehabilitation Services, Cont.

Room 3132
Washington, D.C. 20202-2319
This guide provides basic information on the variety and general scope of federal support and services.

Partial List of Fibromyalgia Researchers

This is just a partial list of individuals and institutions involved in research on fibromyalgia. There are many others interested in fibromyalgia, but this list includes only those whose work has been published in medical journals. For information on these physicians' policies for accepting new patients, contact the rheumatology or psychiatric clinic or the office of the individual listed. Most of the physicians are affiliated with a school of medicine but may also have a separate practice at a clinic or hospital, which is also listed if that information was available. The Arthritis Foundation also lists some of the facilities that receive funding for arthritis research and that are currently conducting research on fibromyalgia.

ALABAMA
Laurence A. Bradley, Ph.D.
Associate Professor of Psychology
    and Medicine
University of Alabama-Birmingham
Birmingham, Alabama

CALIFORNIA
P. Kahler Hench, M.D.
F.A.C.P.
Senior Consultant
Division of Rheumatology
Scripps Clinic and Research
    Foundation
10666 North Torrey Pines Road
La Jolla, California

Daniel J. Wallace, M.D.
Associate Clinical Professor of
    Medicine
Department of Medicine
Division of Rheumatology
Cedars-Sinai Medical Center
UCLA School of Medicine
Los Angeles, California

Xavier J. Caro, M.D.
Associate Clinical Professor of
    Medicine
University of California
Los Angeles, California
Northridge Hospital Medical Center
Northridge, California

ILLINOIS

Muhammad B. Yunus, M.D.
Assistant Professor of Medicine
Division of Rheumatology
Department of Medicine
University of Illinois
College of Medicine at Peoria
P.O. Box 1649
Peoria, Illinois

KANSAS

Frederick Wolfe, M.D.
Clinical Professor of Medicine
University of Kansas
School of Medicine
Director, Wichita Arthritis Center
1035 North Emporia, #230
Wichita, Kansas

LOUISIANA

Dennis W. Boulware, M.D.
Chief, Section of Rheumatology
Tulane University Medical Center
1430 Tulane Avenue
New Orleans, Louisiana

MASSACHUSETTS

Don L. Goldenberg, M.D.
Professor of Medicine
Tufts University School of Medicine
Boston, Massachusetts
Chief of Rheumatology
Director, Arthritis-Fibrositis Clinic
Newton-Wellesley Hospital
2014 West Washington Street
Newton, Massachusetts

David T. Felson, M.D., MPH
Associate Professor of Medicine
A203 Boston University School of
    Medicine
80 East Concord Street
Boston, Massachusetts

James Hudson, M.D.
Associate Professor of Psychiatry
Harvard Medical School
Boston, Massachusetts
Associate Chief
    Biological Psychiatry Laboratory
Laboratories for Psychiatric
    Research and Psychosis Program
McLean Hospital
Belmont, Massachusetts

Harrison G. Pope, Jr., M.D.
Associate Professor of Psychiatry
Harvard Medical School
Boston, Massachusetts
Chief, Biological Psychiatry
    Laboratory
Laboratories for Psychiatric
    Research and Psychosis Program
McLean Hospital
Belmont, Massachusetts

MINNESOTA

Jeffrey M. Thompson, M.D.
Department of Physical Medicine
    and Rehabilitation
Mayo Clinic
Rochester, Minnesota

MISSOURI

John M. Uveges, Ph.D.
Psychology Service
University of Missouri
Columbia School of Medicine
Columbia, Missouri
Psychology Service
Harry S. Truman Memorial Veterans
    Hospital
800 Hospital Drive
Columbia, Missouri

NORTH CAROLINA

Daniel Hamaty, M.D.
Demas Neurology and Medical
  Rehabilitation PA
2115 East 7th Street
Charlotte, North Carolina

OREGON

Robert M. Bennett, M.D., F.R.C.P.,
  F.A.C.P.
Professor of Medicine
Director, Division of Arthritis and
  Rheumatic Diseases
The Oregon Health Sciences
  University
Portland, Oregon

Stephen M. Campbell, M.D.
Associate Professor of Medicine
Division of Arthritis and Rheumatic
  Diseases
The Oregon Health Sciences
  University
Chief, Rheumatology Section
Portland Veterans Administration
Medical Center
Portland, Oregon

PENNSYLVANIA

Dennis C. Turk, Ph.D.
Professor of Psychiatry and
  Anesthesiology
University of Pittsburgh
Pittsburgh, Pennsylvania
Director, Pain Evaluation and
  Treatment Institute
Baum Boulevard at Craig Street
Pittsburg, Pennsylvania

TENNESSEE

Theodore Pincus, M.D.
Division of Rheumatology and
  Immunology
Department of Medicine
Vanderbilt University
  School of Medicine
Nashville, Tennessee

TEXAS

Bernard R. Rubin, D.O., F.A.C.P.,
Professor of Medicine
Chief, Section of Rheumatology
Department of Medicine
Texas College of Osteopathic
  Medicine
Fort Worth, Texas

I. Jon Russell, M.D., Ph.D.
Associate Professor of Medicine
Department of Medicine
Division of Clinical Immunology
University of Texas
Health Science Center at San
  Antonio
7703 Floyd Curl Drive
San Antonio, Texas

WASHINGTON

Martin J. Kushmerick, M.D., Ph.D.
Department of Radiology, SB05
University of Washington
Seattle, Washington

CANADA

Roman Jaeschke, M.D.
St. Joseph's Hospital
Fontbonne Building
50 Charlton Avenue East
Hamilton, Ontario

Harold Merskey, D.M.
Professor of Psychiatry
University of Western Ontario
Director of Research
London Psychiatric Hospital
London, Ontario

Glen A. McCain, M.D., F.R.C.P.
Associate Professor
Department of Medicine
University Hospital
University of Western Ontario
London, Ontario

Harvey Moldofsky, M.D.
Professor, Department of Psychiatry
   and Medicine
University of Toronto
Toronto, Ontario
Toronto Western Hospital
399 Bathurst Street
Toronto, Ontario

W.J. Reynolds, M.D., F.R.C.P.
Rheumatic Disease Unit
Toronto Western Hospital
399 Bathurst Street
Toronto, Ontario

Hugh Smythe, M.D.
Professor and Head
Rheumatic Diseases Unit
The Wellesley Hospital
University of Toronto
160 Wellesley Street East
Toronto, Ontario

Suggested Reading

American Medical Association. *Guide to Prescription and Over-the-Counter Drugs*. New York: Random House, 1988. An excellent overall guide to drugs, including information on side effects, interactions, and special precautions as well as a descriptive listing for more than 2,500 brandname and generic drugs.

Arthritis Foundation. *Understanding Arthritis*. New York: Charles Scribner's Sons, 1984. A general overview of arthritis.

Benson, Herbert, M.D. with Miriam Z. Klipper. *The Relaxation Response*. New York: Random House, 1975. Explains the concept of meditation and provides instructions.

Benson, Herbert, M.D. with William Proctor. *Your Maximum Mind*. New York: Random House, 1987. Shows readers how to tap their inner resources.

Bolles, Richard Nelson. *What Color is Your Parachute?* Berkeley, CA: Ten Speed Press, 1991. An outstanding guide to job-hunting and making career changes. Updated annually.

Brown, Barbara, Ph.D. *Between Health & Illness*. New York: Bantam, 1985. Addresses stress and the nature of well-being.

————. *New Mind, New Body, Bio-Feedback: New Directions for the Mind*. New York, Bantam, 1975. Over 500 pages of information on the concept and use of biofeedback.

Choices: A Sexual Guide for the Physically Disabled. Boston: Spalding Rehabilitation Hospital, 1990.

Comfort, Alex, M.B., Ph.D. 2nd ed. *The Joy of Sex*. New York: Fireside, 1972. Although this is intended to be a general guide to lovemaking, there are sections that could be of help to anyone who has a chronic illness that makes sexual intimacy difficult.

Conan, Susan, Ed.D. *Living with Chronic Fatigue*. Dallas: Taylor Publishing Co., 1990. New strategies for coping with chronic fatigue syndrome and chronic illnesses in general.

Cooper, Kenneth, M.D., M.P.H. *Aerobics*. New York: Bantam, 1968. Explains the concept of aerobic exercises in lay terms and provides an exercise program. Note: Any exercise program should be approved by your doctor.

Cousins, Norman. *Anatomy of an Illness As Perceived by the Patient*. New York: Bantam, 1983. An excellent example of a person taking charge of his illness, the partnership possible between patient and doctor, and the beneficial effects of laughter on health. Highly recommended.

————. *The Healing Heart*. New York: Avon, 1984. Cousins explains how the power of positive emotions prevented him from panicking when he had a major heart attack.

Dachman, Ken and Jon Lyons. *You Can Relieve Pain*. New York: Harper Perennial, 1991. Guide to using imagery to reduce pain.

Davidson, Paul, M.D. *Chronic Muscle Pain Syndrome*. New York: Berkley, 1991. Looks at fibromyalgia but considers stress to be the cause. Indicates that controlling stress will restore you to full health.

Enby, G. *Let There Be Love*. New York: Zebra, 1983.

Ford, Norman. *Sleep Well, Live Well*. New York: Zebra, 1983. Tips on how to get a better night's sleep.

Goldstein, Jay A., M.D. *Could Your Doctor Be Wrong?* New York: Pharos, 1991. An excellent examination of many conditions that are undiagnosed or misdiagnosed, including fibromyalgia.

Guide to Independent Living, for People with Arthritis. Atlanta, GA: Arthritis Foundation, 1988. Write the foundation at 1314 Spring Street, N.W., Atlanta, GA, 30309, to obtain a copy. Over 400 pages of practical tips and resources for people with arthritis. Although mainly for those with rheumatoid arthritis and osteoarthritis, much of its information is valuable to those with FM. It includes the names and addresses of organizations and resources for everything from traveling assistance to adaptive devices to agencies that can provide help. An excellent resource book.

Hastings, K., A.M. Schellen, and V. Verkuyl. *Not Made of Stone: The Sexual Problems of Handicapped People*. Springfield, IL. Charles C. Thomas, 1974.

Jetter, Judy and Nancy Kadlec, O.T.R. *The Arthritis Book of Water Exercise*. New York: Holt, Rinehart, and Winston, 1985. Well-illustrated book of exercises based on the Arthritis Aquatics Program, which is cosponsored by the Arthritis Foundation and the YMCA.

Kievman, Beverly and Susie Blackman. *For Better or for Worse: A Couple's Guide to Dealing with Chronic Illness*. Chicago: Contemporary, 1989. An excellent look at the problems a couple faces when one partner becomes chronically ill.

Kuntzleman, Charles T. and editors of *Consumer Guide*. *The Complete Book of Walking*. New York: Pocket Books, 1982. Covers everything from proper shoes and sensible walking programs to special health problems.

Lorig, Kate, R.N. and James F. Fries, M.D. 3rd ed. *The Arthritis Handbook: A Tested Self-Management Program for Coping with Your Arthritis*. Reading, MA: Addision-Wesley Publishing, 1990. Recommended by the Arthritis Foundation and used in their self-help courses, this book covers the major forms of arthritis, helpful exercises (with illustrations), pain management, problem solving, feelings, nutrition, drugs, and doctors.

Ornstein, Robert and David Sobel. *The Healing Brain: Breakthrough Discoveries About How the Brain Keeps Us Healthy*. New York: Simon and Schuster, 1988. Explains how the brain controls the immune system, regulates pain, and uses our emotions for better health.

Pelletier, Kenneth R. *Mind As Healer—Mind As Slayer: A Holistic Approach to Preventing Stress Disorders*. New York: Delta, 1977. This book defines the role of stress in four major types of illness: cardiovascular disease, cancer, arthritis, and respiratory disease. Although fibromyalgia is not discussed, many of the theories regarding the adverse effects of stress apply to those with fibromyalgia.

Pizele, Sefra Kobrin. *We Are Not Alone: Learning to Live with Chronic Illness*. New York: Workman Publishing, 1986. Although the author has systemic lupus erythematosis, this book is for anyone who has a chronic illness. Highly recommended.

Prudden, Bonnie. *Pain Erasure: The Bonnie Prudden Way*. New York: Ballantine, 1985. An explanation of myotherapy (a form of massage therapy) which may bring some relief to those with FM.

Raley, Patricia E. *Making Love: How to Be Your Own Sex Therapist*. New York: Avon, 1980. This covers not only the expected problems that occur in sexual relationships but also such areas as body image and self-image. Written in plain, straightforward language.

Stern, Bert. 4th ed. *The Pill Book*. New York: Bantam, 1990. An illustrated guide to the drugs most commonly prescribed in the United States.

Task Force on Concerns of Physically Disabled Women. *Toward Intimacy: Family Planning and Sexuality Concerns of Physically Disabled Women*. New York: Human Science Press, 1979.

————. *Within Reach: Providing Family Planning Services to Physically Disabled Women*. New York: Human Sciences Press, 1978.

Westberg, Granger E. *Good Grief: A Constructive Approach to the Problem of Loss*. Philadelphia: Fortress Press, 1985. A Christian approach to coping with the grief caused by loss.

Publications that Were Helpful to the Author

American Journal of Nursing
American Journal of Psychiatry
Archives of Physical Medicine and Rehabilitation
Arthritis and Rheumatism
Arthritis News
Australian Family Physician
British Journal of Rheumatology
Canadian Medical Association Journal
Comprehensive Therapy
Digestive Diseases and Sciences
Hospital Practice
Journal of the American Medical Association
Journal of Behavioral Therapy
Journal of Consulting and Clinical Psychology
Journal of Internal Medicine
Journal of Personal Assessment
Journal of Psychosomatic Research
Journal of Rheumatology
Modern Medicine
Oral Surgery, Oral Medicine, and Oral Pathology
Pain
Patient Care
Pharmacotherapy
Physical Therapy
Psychosomatic Medicine
Scandinavian Journal of Rehabilitation Medicine
The American Journal of Medicine
The Journal of Musculoskeletal Medicine
The Medical Journal of Rehabilitation
The Physician and Sports Medicine